Objective Structured Clinical Examinations

Sondra Zabar • Elizabeth Krajic Kachur
Adina Kalet • Kathleen Hanley
Editors

Objective Structured Clinical Examinations

10 Steps to Planning and Implementing
OSCEs and Other Standardized
Patient Exercises

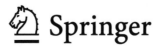 Springer

Editors
Sondra Zabar
Department of Medicine
Division of General Internal Medicine
Section of Primary Care
New York University School of Medicine
New York, NY, USA

Adina Kalet
Department of Medicine
Division of General Internal Medicine
Section of Primary Care
New York University School of Medicine
New York, NY, USA

Elizabeth Krajic Kachur
Medical Education Development
National and International Consulting
New York, NY, USA

Kathleen Hanley
Department of Medicine
Division of General Internal Medicine
Section of Primary Care
New York University School of Medicine
New York, NY, USA

ISBN 978-1-4614-3748-2   ISBN 978-1-4614-3749-9 (eBook)
DOI 10.1007/978-1-4614-3749-9
Springer New York Heidelberg Dordrecht London

Library of Congress Control Number: 2012951673

Foreword

In the late 1960s, as a clinical teacher and examiner, I was faced with a dilemma. The final clinical examination in the UK was a high-stakes test, success in which was necessary for the student to graduate with a medical degree. The approach, however, had come under increased scrutiny and had been recognized as unreliable and criticized because it sampled only limited areas of clinical competence. Similar criticisms had been made of written examinations in the form of essay questions, and MCQs had been introduced because of their greater reliability and the more extensive sample of knowledge assessed. It appeared to me that the ability to answer an MCQ correctly did not necessarily indicate that the student had the necessary skills to become a good doctor. Essential was some form of assessment of clinical competence. The objective structured clinical examination (OSCE) was developed as a flexible approach, which made possible the assessment of a wide range of clinical skills more objectively than had been possible in the past.

The approach proved attractive to teachers, examiners, curriculum developers, educationalists, and students and over the following 40 years became the gold standard for the assessment of clinical competence. Over these years, more than 1,000 papers have been published on the OSCE and considerable experience and understanding has been gained as to the learning outcomes that can be assessed, the purposes for which an OSCE can be used, how small and large groups of students can be examined in a wide range of settings, how the examination should be planned and set up, the roles of the examiners, the different approaches to the use of patients including standardized patients, the types of stations created, how the OSCE can be scored and standards specified, and how feedback can be provided to students.

Many books have been published describing OSCE examinations in a range of specialties, assessing a spectrum of learning outcomes. There is a need, however, for a text such as this book that provides the teacher and student new to the subject with an overview of the approaches, while at the same time conveying an understanding of the basic underpinning principles implicit in an OSCE and how these are reflected in an OSCE as implemented in practice. The text has been carefully crafted and will also be of value to the more experienced examiner, increasing their appreciation of the approach and how maximum gains can be obtained from its use.

With moves to outcome-based education and competency-based assessment, more personalized and adaptive learning, greater use of educational technology including simulations, and demands for more authenticity in learning and assessment, the OSCE will maintain its position as an important assessment tool alongside other approaches including portfolios and work-based assessment tools. The assessment of competence in the health care student or professional is almost certainly the most important responsibility facing the teacher or trainer and indeed of all health care professionals. Drs. Zabar, Kachur, Hanley, and Kalet's ten steps to planning and implementing OSCEs and other standardized patient exercises should enable them to undertake this duty effectively and efficiently.

Dundee, UK   Ronald M. Harden, OBE, MD, FRCP (Glas), FRCS (Ed), FRCPC

Preface

This book is a practical manual for educators in the health professions wishing to build a state-of-the-art performance assessment program for their trainees.

Why make the considerable investment required to do this well? Why go through the trouble of choosing competencies to measure, writing and piloting cases, recruiting and training standardized patients (SPs), developing standards, and scheduling hoards of students into countless 15-min rotation slots many times a year? Simply, there is no better method to measure the areas of expertise our patients rely on and expect their health care providers to have. Clinical knowledge, although it can be reliably and validly tested through multiple-choice exams, does not translate directly into clinical skill. Because the health professions student must learn to integrate and apply their knowledge, as well as communication, professionalism, ethical, reasoning, and physical examination skills, Objective Structured Clinical Examinations (OSCEs), which simulate—physically and emotionally—the actual physician–patient encounter, are needed.

This book started as a handout to accompany a highly successful workshop at the Association for Program Directors in Internal Medicine annual meeting on developing SP programs. Attendees suggested useful expansions and encouraged its publication. They also made us realize that while the justification for developing SP exercises in physician training had already been argued, there were no available resources on how to design OSCE cases, how to recruit and train SPs, managing logistics, and all the nitty-gritty things that make an SP program sing or sag. This book is meant to fill that gap.

The editors and authors of this book are my partners in building and leading the NYU/Bellevue Primary Care Residency Program, and they are in a good position to create such a manual because of their extensive experience, dedication, and pioneering scholarship in medical education. Beginning modestly in the late 1980s we experimented with SP encounters in our doctoring course for medical students and in the Primary Care Internal Medicine Residency Program. By 2000, we had begun to use SPs for formative and summative educational experiences on a large scale and across a broad range of training levels and content areas including geriatrics, women's and immigrant health, and addiction medicine. We next gained experience in creating research-quality OSCEs to assess communication skills training, first in the multi-institutional Macy Initiative in Health Communication project (medical students) and then in a disaster preparedness project on psychosocial aspects of bioterroism jointly funded by the Centers for Disease Control and the Association for American Medical Colleges (physicians, nurse practitioners, and physician assistants). We also developed complimentary baseline and end-of-third-year medical student clinical encounter skills assessments to allow us to understand how clinical skills progress in novice health care providers. In the mid 2000s we began to pilot the use of unannounced SPs in our residency program in order to understand how what we measure in OSCEs translates to the real practice setting. Currently, our medical students encounter upwards of 40 SP cases during medical school; our primary care residents, 45 in 3 years of training. These encounters range from formative exercises designed purely for learning purposes, which include immediate feedback and extensive debriefing, to summative, high-stakes exams. The experiences provide opportunities to test multiple dimensions (e.g., preparation, communication, clinical reasoning, time management, preventive medicine, error prevention, and management) of good doctoring and approach the complexities of real patients and the stresses of actual clinical practice in a controlled setting.

After some initial resistance to the idea of OSCEs, our students and residents early on expressed their appreciation for the opportunity to practice difficult tasks in a safe environment. Now, although some students still get nervous about them, OSCEs are highly popular and are perceived as valuable teaching tools. Our residents by and large rate them consistently highly and feel they are an efficient use of time and an excellent learning experience. Faculty who participate in OSCEs—developing cases, observing and giving feedback, debriefing—report benefitting greatly from the opportunity to directly observe and calibrate their expectations of trainees. Clinical leadership appreciates that we are rigorously addressing important issues such as communication, patient safety, and patient activation. And the many actors working closely with us in this endeavor feel that they are engaged in highly meaningful work, both personally and professionally. In the Primary Care Internal Medicine Residency Program, our annual day-long OSCE is not only a central feature of program evaluation and resident assessment but has also become an important community-building experience for residents, staff, and faculty.

OSCEs are now used in the training of most health professionals in the USA and elsewhere. They are used to assess knowledge, skills, professionalism, ethical behavior, physical examination skills, and the ability to work with difficult patients, with diverse cultural backgrounds, with patients on the phone, and with families. They can measure simple processes (does the learner recommend stopping smoking) and very complex ones (does the novice have the professional maturity to manage telling the non-English speaking family member about an unexpected death, through an interpreter, and ask for an autopsy).

So much progress has been made in our ability to ensure that we graduate physicians capable of practicing medicine in a rapidly evolving health care environment. And yet so much is yet to be done. New curriculum needs are emerging every year—interprofessional education, patient safety, systems-based practice, informatics, disaster medicine, to name a few recent additions. We have found that having a rich and flexible SP-based OSCE program has allowed us to meet these new curriculum and assessment challenges in a rigorous and exciting way. Developing and implementing an OSCE is a highly creative and scholarly activity, which requires a group of educators to do the difficult work of coming to a consensus on educational priorities and setting standards for trainee performance. The process is scholarly because, when engaging in OSCE development, one cannot avoid unearthing important unanswered questions about health professional competence and training. Many of these questions can even be answered with OSCEs. For all these reasons we find this work enjoyable and intellectually engaging. In this book, Drs. Zabar, Kachur, Hanley, and Kalet share with you our hard-earned experience so that you can avoid many of the pitfalls and get to the fun and meaningful stuff more directly. Call us, come visit, come see OSCEs in action, and organize a workshop. We stand ready to help.

New York, NY

Mack Lipkin, MD

Acknowledgments

First of all, we must thank the thousands of NYU medical students who have participated in OSCEs over the past decade as well the hundreds of NYU School of Medicine residents and chief residents—from Primary Care, Categorical Medicine, Surgery, Orthopedics, Anesthesiology, OB/GYN—who trusted that the SP exercises we introduced would be educational and relevant. We are immensely grateful to our many creative and dedicated colleagues on the NYUSOM General Internal Medicine/Primary Care faculty in addition to this book's contributors, who wrote cases, observed and evaluated learners, trained countless SPs, and conducted faculty development: especially, David Stevens, Jennifer Adams, Richard Greene, Robert Caldwell, David Coun, Leslie Cheung, Judith Su, and Carrie Mahowald. Special thanks are due to Ellen Pearlman and Judith Brenner, who designed the workshop that included the first incarnation of this manual. We are also indebted to Michael Yedidia for the initial formulation of our OSCE checklist. Martin Lischka of the Medical University of Vienna, Charlotte Leanderson and colleagues at the Karolinska Institute, and Erik Langenau of the National Board of Osteopathic Medical Examiners graciously read later drafts of the manuscript and each provided invaluable feedback for improvement. Over the years, the success of each OSCE we have conducted has been thanks to our organizational gurus: the inimitable Marian Anderson, Amy Hsieh, Regina Richter, Julianne Cameron, Lindsey Disney, Ivey Overstreet, and Katherine Miller. Ari Kreith, who has cast and directed hundreds of SPs for our programs over the past decade, deserves an Oscar. We are incredibly fortunate to work at institutions who value the importance of provider education to patient care—Gouverneur Healthcare Services, Bellevue Hospital Center, and NYUSOM and its Office of Medical Education, all of whom supported this overall project with donated space and other resources from day one. Finally, we would like to thank the many standardized patients who have partnered with us to change medical education.

Contents

Contributors

Lynn Buckvar-Keltz, MD Office of Student Affairs, New York University School of Medicine, New York, NY, USA

Angela Burgess Program for Medical Education Innovations and Research, New York University School of Medicine, New York, NY, USA

Colleen C. Gillespie, PhD Department of Medicine, Division of General Internal Medicine, New York University School of Medicine, New York, NY, USA

Kathleen Hanley, MD Department of Medicine, Division of General Internal Medicine, Section of Primary Care, New York University School of Medicine, New York, NY, USA

Ronald M. Harden Association of Medical Education in Europe (AMEE), Dundee, Scotland, UK

Julia Hyland Bruno Program for Medical Education Innovations and Research, New York University School of Medicine, New York, NY, USA

Elizabeth Krajic Kachur, PhD Medical Education Development, National and International Consulting, New York, NY, USA

Adina Kalet, MD, MPH Department of Medicine, Division of General Internal Medicine, Section of Primary Care, New York University School of Medicine, New York, NY, USA

Mack Lipkin, MD Department of Medicine, Division of General Internal Medicine, Section of Primary Care, New York University School of Medicine, New York, NY, USA

Jennifer Ogilvie, MD, FACS Department of Surgery, New York University School of Medicine, New York, NY, USA

Barbara Porter, MD, MPH Department of Medicine, Bellevue Hospital Center, New York, NY, USA

Linda Tewksbury, MD Department of Pediatrics, New York University School of Medicine, New York, NY, USA

Sandra Yingling, PhD Office of Medical Education, New York University School of Medicine, New York, NY, USA

Sondra Zabar, MD Department of Medicine, Division of General Internal Medicine, Section of Primary Care, New York University School of Medicine, New York, NY, USA

Introduction

Sondra Zabar, Elizabeth Krajic Kachur, Kathleen Hanley, and Adina Kalet

How to Use this Book

Creating objective structured clinical exams (OSCEs) or other standardized patient (SP) exercises can feel overwhelming, but the benefits of this kind of practice-based learning and assessment—for future health care practitioners and their future patients!—make them work definitely worth doing. This is why we wrote this book. It is our hope that the systematic approach offered here will make it easier for more people to get involved in the process of creating OSCEs or similar SP exercises. Using a road map like the one contained in Chap. 2 (our "Ten Steps"), the process is really quite doable as well as rewarding.

SPs and OSCEs play an increasing role within contemporary health professions education across all disciplines and across the continuum of training. They are important educational tools for high-quality teaching (formative assessments) as well as for the evaluation of basic and advanced clinical skills (summative assessments). Program evaluations increasingly include OSCEs to measure the impact of curricular interventions.

Licensing and accrediting organizations around the world have embraced OSCEs and SPs. For example, the Accreditation Council for Graduate Medical Education (ACGME) in the United States has recommended them as key components of their assessment Toolbox (ACGME/ ABMS Joint Initiative 2000). The US National Board of Medical Examiners (NBME) implements OSCE-type assessments as part of licensure (www.usmle.org/step-2-cs/). Efforts such as these enable health professions educators to better fulfill their obligations to society.

Though many institutions have access to a sophisticated clinical skills center, many do not. We wrote this book based on our 20-year experience producing OSCEs without a clinical skills center—in empty classrooms or walk-in clinics on weekends, using well-trained actors and carefully designed clinical scenarios. Our experience covers a broad range of multidisciplinary and inter-professional collaborations. Through this work we have fine-tuned our approach to designing and implementing successful OSCEs. No matter how small or large your group of learners, this book can help you do the same. While OSCEs are resource-intensive endeavors, the benefits to all involved make the investment well-leveraged.

Organizing an OSCE is a major undertaking and, as with most other educational projects, requires strong and committed leadership. Many individuals are needed for planning, preparation, implementation, and evaluation. The production of a successful OSCE may result in a powerful synergy capable of invigorating educational programs. The event itself brings together faculty, learners, and staff to put their efforts towards a common goal. OSCEs produce meaningful experiences and useful data. Despite the stresses and risks involved, most people leave the event recognizing the value and feeling enriched.

In the rest of this chapter, we define key terms and review the history of OSCEs and SP programs and their current applications. Chapter 2 provides a detailed, comprehensive ten-step approach to the process of OSCE design and implementation. Each section concludes with a list of best practices or guidelines. Chapters 3 and 4 are devoted to emerging issues. Good OSCE data predictably identify and indicate strategies for helping learners in need of remediation, as surveyed in Chap. 3. Looking beyond the training context, Chap. 4 explores how demands for more "in vivo"

S. Zabar, M.D. (✉) • K. Hanley, M.D. • A. Kalet, M.D., M.P.H.
Department of Medicine, Division of General Internal Medicine, Section of Primary Care, New York University School of Medicine, 550 First Avenue, BCD D401, New York, NY 10016, USA
e-mail: sondra.zabar@nyumc.org

E.K. Kachur, Ph.D.
Medical Education Development, National and International Consulting, 201 East 21st Street, New York, NY 10016, USA

S. Zabar et al. (eds.), *Objective Structured Clinical Examinations*, DOI 10.1007/978-1-4614-3749-9_1, © Springer Science+Business Media New York 2013

assessment can be met through the use and implementation of incognito or unannounced SPs (USPs) in clinical settings. The Appendices at the back of this book contain blank versions of all the forms and worksheets included in the main text, sample OSCE cases and checklists, and suggested further resources.

Definitions

Standardized patients (SPs) are individuals who portray a specific clinical case in a consistent. Typically they are not afflicted by the bio-psychosocial conditions they are depicting. Rather, they are simulating clinical problems solely for the purpose of training and assessment. When SPs were introduced to medical education by Howard Barrows in 1963 they were called "programmed" patients (Barrows and Abrahamson 1964) to reflect the educator's ability to shape the scenarios in order to meet curriculum or assessment needs. In the 1980s the term "simulated patient" became popular. With increasing use in assessment and the corresponding need for controlling the test stimulus, "standardized patient" is often times the preferred term, especially in North America.

Objective structured clinical exams or exercises (OSCEs) are training or assessment programs in which learners rotate through a series of time-limited "stations." In encounters with SPs in each (or most) of a series of stations, the learner is asked to perform specific tasks that are kept constant across all trainees. Rating forms with predetermined performance criteria are used to assess the learner's performance in a standardized fashion. Figure 1.1 illustrates the SP cases a learner might encounter in a ten-station OSCE.

History and Current Use of SPs and OSCEs

In 1963 Howard Barrows, then at the University of Southern California in Los Angeles, hired a healthy woman to simulate the case of a paraplegic patient with multiple sclerosis for his neurology clerkship students. This was the introduction of SPs into medical education (Barrows and Abrahamson 1964). Beginning in the early 1970s Paula Stillman, then at the University of Arizona, used simulated mothers for teaching interviewing skills. She also created the Arizona Clinical Interview Rating Scale (ACIR) (Stillman et al. 1977) which is still used in some OSCEs today. Barrows and Stillman can

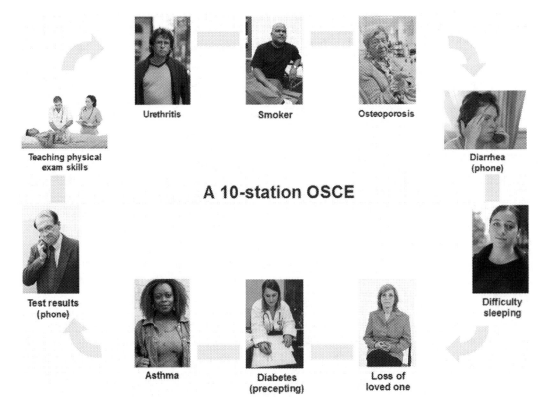

Fig. 1.1 A ten-station OSCE: Circuit of SP scenarios (i.e., stations) through which learners rotate

be considered the originators of a worldwide movement to use SPs in health professions education.

In 1992, the Association of American Medical Colleges (AAMC) organized a national consensus conference on SPs (Anderson and Kassebaum 1993). Since then, the field has expanded further and standards of practice have developed for the use of SPs (Adamo 2003). In 2001 the Association of Standardized Patient Educators (ASPE) was formed, creating an international network of professionals devoted to SP work and research. Annual conferences, an active listserv, and an extensive Web site (www.aspeducators.org) offer the opportunity to exchange resources (e.g., cases, SP contact information, references, moulage techniques to simulate physical signs) and to develop best practice guidelines.

OSCEs originated in Dundee, Scotland, in the early 1970s. Ronald Harden (see the Foreword of this book) and his colleagues published the first article describing these multiple station exams (Harden et al. 1975). By September 1983, Emil Petrusa and his colleagues at the University of Texas Medical Branch (UTMB) in Galveston, TX mounted the first such exam for about 140 Internal Medicine clerkship students. It consisted of 17 station pairs, a total of 34 stations, each 4 min in length. The project was presented at the annual AAMC meeting in the fall of 1984 (Petrusa et al. 1984). Two years later, in the spring of 1986, one of this book's coeditors (Kachur, then at Albert Einstein College of Medicine) organized the first OSCE in the New York City area. Other early adopters in the United States included Southern Illinois University (SIU) and the University of Massachusetts (UMass). Worldwide there were many countries which held their first OSCEs in the late 1970s and early 1980s. These include Canada, Australia, The Netherlands, Ireland, Sweden, and South Africa.

In the 1990s, The Macy Foundation funded a national consortium of six regional consortia that embraced a total of 28 US medical schools in an effort to promote performance-based testing. The initiative resulted in the publications of some 30 articles (e.g., Morrison and Barrows 1998; Yedidia et al. 2003) that advanced the field in areas such as case and rating form development and scoring, exam impact on the curriculum, SP performance quality control, and SP versus faculty observers.

Also in the early 1990s, the Educational Commission for Foreign Medical Graduates (ECFMG) developed a growing interest in performance-based assessment to assure adequate clinical competence and English proficiency of international medical graduates (IMGs). This led to extensive pilot testing that further expanded the field (e.g., Sutnick et al. 1993). By 1998 the ECFMG had created a secure assessment center in Philadelphia, PA and fully implemented its Clinical Skills Assessment (CSA) as a requirement for all IMGs who wanted to take up postgraduate training in the United States. Six years later, in 2004, the NBOME followed suit and opened five testing centers around the country. Since then all US medical graduates and all IMGs are mandated to complete Step 2 Clinical Skills (CS) of the US Medical Licensing Examination (USMLE; www.usmle.org/step-2-cs/). The National Board of Osteopathic Medical Examiners (NBOME) administered its first Comprehensive Osteopathic Medical Licensing Examination Level 2—Performance Evaluation (COMLEX-USA Level 2-PE, www.nbome.org/comlex-pe.asp?m=can) in also 2004. The first Medical Council of Canada Qualifying Examination Part II (MCCQE Part II, www.mcc.ca/en/exams/qe2/), by contrast, was held in 1992 (Boulet et al. 2009). Table 1.1 compares key features of the USMLE Step 2 CS, COMLEX-USA Level 2-PE, and MCCQE Part II, three largely compatible licensing OSCEs.

Overall, the United States has not been one of the early adopters of OSCE methodologies. For example, the Canadian Certification in Family Medicine nationwide licensing exam (www.cfpc.ca/FMExam/) was initiated already in 1970 (Lamont and Hennen 1972) and was delivered in English and French from the start. Since OSCEs originated in the UK, Commonwealth connections and United Nations grants fostered the initial dissemination around the globe. Hence the interesting journey of the OSCEs to the United States via Canada. For a more extensive history of the OSCE, readers can explore Brian Hodges' (2009) social history of the exam, which explores how discourses of performance, psychometrics, and production have propelled the development of this educational method.

Many training programs worldwide are now using SPs and OSCEs extensively as a summative assessment of learner competence, and increasingly programs use OSCEs to measure the effect of their curricular interventions. OSCEs have even been introduced as an admissions screening tool (Harris 2011). Many content areas have been addressed with the help of OSCEs. These include complex communication, physical exam, and procedural skills such as cultural competence (Zabar et al. 2006; Aeder et al. 2007; Altshuler & Kachur 2001), genetics (Altshuler et al. 2008), gastroenterology (Chander et al. 2009), substance abuse (Parish et al. 2006), and teaching skills (Zabar et al. 2004). In combination with other assessments, SPs and OSCEs allow programs to both educate and assess learners, ensuring clinical competence (Kachur 2007).

How Can SPs and OSCEs Satisfy National Competency Guidelines?

As Table 1.2 illustrates, each individual OSCE station can address multiple competency assessments in Undergraduate, Graduate, and Continuing Medical Education. Over the last few years there has been a clear movement to accept the ACGME Core Competencies (2001) as the standard for the entire continuum of medical education in the United States. Other countries have developed similar competency

Table 1.1 US and Canadian Performance-based Licensure Exams (administered towards the end of medical school or within the first postgraduate year)

Exam name	Year initiated	National Administration	OSCE structure	Key domains	Scoring and reporting
USMLE Step 2 CS (United States Medical Licensing Examination Step 2 Clinical Skills)	2004	• Year-round • 5 regional test centers • Center-based SP trainers and SPs • Multiple test versions	• 12 graded stations + ? exploratory stations • 15 min encounters + 15 min patient note writing • SPs rate encounters, physician raters for patient note	1. Integrated clinical encounter (i.e., history taking, physical exam, documentation) 2. Communication and interpersonal skills (information gathering/sharing, establishing rapport) 3. English proficiency	• Each candidate must to pass each domain
COMLEX-USA Level 2-PE (Comprehensive Osteopathic Medical Licensing Examination Level 2—Performance Evaluation)[a]	2004	• Year-round • 1 national test center • Center-based SP trainers and SPs • Multiple test versions	• 12 graded stations + 2 exploratory stations • 14 min encounters + 9 min written patient note • SP raters for encounters, physician raters for post-encounter notes and OMT (via video tape)	1. Doctor–patient communication and professionalism 2. Data gathering (i.e., history taking, physical exam) 3. Documentation and synthesis of findings 4. Osteopathic principles and OMT	• Station scores are compensatory but candidates must pass the Humanism (SP-only ratings) plus the Biomedical/Biomechanical domains (SP and physician ratings)
MCCQE Part II (Medical Council of Canada Qualifying Examination Part II)	1992	• Spring and fall • Multiple university-based test sites • Local SP trainers and SPs • Multiple test versions	• 12 graded stations + 2 exploratory stations • 10 min encounters or 5 min encounter + 5 min written task • Physician rater in room	1. Data gathering (i.e., history taking, physical exam) 2. Patient interaction 3. Problem solving and decision making 4. Legal, ethical, and organizational issues	• Each station has equal value • Criterion-referenced

[a]Osteopathic medicine (not to be confused with chiropractic) is equivalent to allopathic medicine except that it focuses more on primary care, neuromusculoskeletal causes of disease and it includes osteopathic manipulation treatment (OMT) (see www.aacom.org for more information)

Table 1.2 Potential coverage of national and international competency standards through OSCE stations (adapted from Kachur 2007)

Potential SP or station scenarios	Health advocate	Communicator	Professional	Scholar	Manager	Collaborator
Undergraduate medical education (AAMC Medical School Objectives Project 1998)	Physicians must be skillful		Physicians must be altruistic	Physicians must be knowledgeable	Physicians must be dutiful	
Graduate Medical Education (ACGME 2001)	Patient care	Interpersonal and communication skills	Professionalism	Medical knowledge	Practice-based learning and improvement	System-based practice
Continuing Medical Education (IOM 2003)	Provide patient-centered care			Employ evidence-based practice	Apply quality improvement; utilize informatics	Work in interdisciplinary teams
International Standards (Royal College of Physicians and Surgeons of Canada 2005)	Health advocate	Communicator	Professional	Scholar	Manager	Collaborator
Initial work-up of patient with undifferentiated problem (e.g., fatigue, cough)	X	X	X	X		X
Prevention counseling (e.g., smoking cessation, immunization)	X	X	X	X		X
Discuss management of chronic disease with patient	X	X	X	X		X
Telephone follow-up of lab results (e.g., cholesterol test, PPD)	X	X	X	X		X
Chart review (e.g., discuss chart note indicating medical error with colleague)	X	X	X	X	X	X
Precept a medical trainee (e.g., physical diagnosis, patient management)	X	X	X	X	X	
Perform an online literature search and discuss findings with a patient	X	X	X	X	X	X

The table suggests how the AAMC Learning Objectives for Medical Student Education, the ACGME Core Competencies, the IOM Competencies Required of All Health Care Professionals, and the six overlapping roles of the Medical Expert in the CanMEDS Physician Competency Framework can be aligned and specifies some SP scenarios suitable for assessing each competency

frameworks and OSCEs are frequently mentioned as an efficient and effective teaching or assessment tool.

CanMEDs is the model that was developed by the Royal College of Physicians and Surgeons of Canada. The CanMEDs model originated in 1996 and was updated in 2005. It envisions the responsibilities of physicians as a collection of six core roles which together characterize the Medical Expert: Communicator, Collaborator, Manager, Health Advocate, Scholar and Professional (Royal College of Physicians and Surgeons of Canada 2005). Its popularity has gone way beyond the Canadian borders. Over the years various OSCE reports have plotted stations against this framework (e.g., Jefferies et al. 2007; also see Table 1.2 for an illustration of how the CanMEDs roles are compatible with other accepted competency frameworks).

In Europe the latest effort to harmonize medical education includes the two-level Tuning Project (Medicine) for undergraduate medical education, which specifies 12 core Outcomes expected of all medical school graduates, regardless of what European country they are from, as well as specific performance Competencies which can easily be assessed in OSCE stations (Cumming and Ross 2008).

Worldwide there are efforts underway to transform time-based education (i.e., requiring a certain length of training in terms of months or years) into competency-based education (i.e., requiring the demonstration of specific competencies as requirement for promotion). Since OSCEs are capable of assessing many core competencies regardless of the framework utilized, they are likely to become an even more prominent assessment tools in the future.

Elizabeth Krajic Kachur, Sondra Zabar, Kathleen Hanley,
Adina Kalet, Julia Hyland Bruno, and Colleen C. Gillespie

Step 1

Identify Available Resources

Assemble a Team

Objective structured clinical examinations (OSCEs) and other SP projects can be a major undertaking, and as with most other educational projects, collaboration within and across specialties, even across disciplines can only enrich the process. While it is necessary to have strong leaders who believe in the benefits of such comprehensive assessment programs, many other individuals are needed for adequate planning, preparation, and implementation. Table 2.1 details the different roles that OSCEs typically require. Some people may be able to hold multiple roles (e.g., SP and rater) and some roles may be shared among several individuals (e.g., co-leadership). There will be a need for a "core team" (e.g., OSCE committee) that is responsible for planning and

E.K. Kachur, Ph.D.
Medical Education Development,
National and International Consulting,
New York, NY, USA

S. Zabar, M.D. (✉) • K. Hanley, M.D. • A. Kalet, M.D., M.P.H.
Department of Medicine, Division of General Internal Medicine,
Section of Primary Care, New York University School of Medicine,
550 First Avenue, BCD D401, New York, NY 10016, USA
e-mail: sondra.zabar@nyumc.org

J.H. Bruno
Program for Medical Education Innovations and Research,
New York University School of Medicine, New York, NY, USA

C.C. Gillespie, Ph.D.
Department of Medicine, Division of General Internal Medicine,
New York University School of Medicine,
New York, NY, USA

development in advance of the OSCE dates. Participating in such a team provides an opportunity to engage young, upcoming, enthusiastic faculty. Others may be involved only in the implementation phase of the OSCE (e.g., raters). Regularly scheduled meetings can help the committee become more established. After the actual OSCE, the group can work on data interpretation and dissemination.

For those involved in the actual OSCE implementation the most basic job requirements are availability, interest in the project, and stamina. Two additional characteristics of great importance are precision and flexibility. Since OSCEs strive for standardization, it is necessary for all involved to be committed to keeping factors such as timing or case portrayal as consistent as possible. On the other hand, when dealing with large-scale events that involve so many people simultaneously, irregularities are likely to occur (e.g., a learner enters the wrong station, a rater arrives late). Thus, being flexible and willing to adapt is equally important.

It will not always be possible to find all the necessary players within your immediate work area. Thus one should consider looking outside one's division and forging alliances across departments and levels of education (medical school, postgraduate education, continuing medical education). Much of what is required for a successful OSCE is independent of specialty or profession.

Identify Location

When planning where to hold an OSCE, one first needs to decide how important the authenticity of the clinical environment is for the educational exercise at hand. Clinic rooms are of course the ideal spaces for OSCE stations, and one can consider scheduling the OSCE during the weekend or other time when the clinic is closed. OSCE organizers will need to work with clinical administrators well in advance, and also

Table 2.1 OSCE staffing needs (roles needed to run a smooth assessment program)

Roles	Key characteristics	# Needed
Leader	■ Strong motivation to develop and implement project ■ Well connected to procure resources, including access to institutional or local clinical skills testing facilities ■ Involved in medical school curriculum decision-making ■ Able to communicate well and create a team spirit	One or more
Planner	■ Understands logistics of implementing OSCEs ■ Is familiar with local conditions ■ Can entertain multiple options for solving problems	One or more
Administrator	■ Can implement OSCE-related tasks (e.g., scheduling, SP recruitment, photocopying of station materials, data entry) ■ Able to communicate well and create a team spirit ■ Good at troubleshooting and problem solving	One or more (depending on scope)
Station Developer	■ Has relevant clinical experience ■ Is familiar with performance standards ■ Accepts editing	One or more (depending on scope)
Trainer	■ Understands SP and rater roles and case requirements ■ Has teaching skills (e.g., provides constructive feedback) and can manage psychosocial impact of case portrayals ■ Able to communicate well and create a team spirit	One or more (depending on scope)
SPs	■ Committed to standardization of their case portrayal (i.e., not expressing their personal creativity) ■ Comfortable enacting their particular medical case (i.e., not getting emotionally over-involved) ■ Interested in taking on "educational" responsibilities	At least one per station, consider cross-trained alternates
Rater	■ Clear about OSCE goals and performance standards ■ Committed to fair performance assessments (e.g., understands personal rater style and biases) ■ Effective feedback provider (if learners receive post-encounter feedback)	At least one per station, consider cross-covering alternates
Timer	■ Committed to maintaining the OSCE schedule ■ Able to focus despite periods of inactivity (e.g., when learners are in their stations) and distracters (e.g., conversations with faculty on break)	At least one (may not be needed if institution has a dedicated clinical skills center)
Monitor	■ Able to direct rotation flow ■ Can troubleshoot and problem solve (e.g., faculty missing in station, lack of rating forms, video equipment problems)	At least one (may not be needed if institution has a dedicated clinical skills center)
Data Manager	■ Can enter performance data ■ Understands OSCE process ■ Committed to accuracy	At least one
Data Analyst	■ Understands OSCE process ■ Has psychometric skills ■ Understands end-users of results (e.g., learners, program)	At least one
Program Evaluator	■ Understands OSCE process ■ Is familiar with evaluation models (e.g., pre/posttesting) ■ Can develop and analyze program evaluations (e.g., surveys, focus groups)	At least one

take into account technical details such as transport and set-up of props and station materials (e.g., hospital gowns, rating forms, video cameras). Some institutions are fortunate enough to have simulation centers or other dedicated training space with mock examination rooms and built-in monitoring and recording capacities. The OSCE organizer should keep in mind, however, that verisimilitude is not always necessary and learning can also be done in any classroom.

Identify Sources of Funding and Support

There are many venues to explore for funding SP activities and pilot programs. Begin by investigating your own institution's medical education resources at the level of the dean's office, department, and division. There may be funds available that can be used to support OSCEs. In addition, some SP programs have been funded by local medical societies, foundations (e.g., through grants for improving doctor–patient communication), and philanthropic donations.

Best Practices: Assembling a Team

- Establish a clear common goal.
- Build a team with a variety of skills.
- Schedule regular meetings to build group identity.
- Create a common repository (i.e., shared drive, secure Website) for meeting minutes, materials, and protocols.
- Look broadly for suitable sites and funding sources.

Step 2

Agree on Goals and Timeline

Once the decision is made to organize an OSCE, further details need to be worked out. A worksheet such as that shown in Fig. 2.1 (also included in blank form as Appendix A

at the back of this book) can assist with this task. It is often necessary to balance educational opportunities with available resources and strategic considerations.

Figure 2.2 provides a list of core OSCE budget items, filled in for the same example General Internal Medicine Residency OSCE introduced in Fig. 2.1. A blank version of this budget form is also included as Appendix B to assist readers in making cost and resource projections. With most projects funding will be of concern. However, there are various ways to manage with fewer resources (Poenaru et al. 1997; Reznick et al. 1993).

Generally one is wise to start small, and then expand to more complex and ambitious training or assessment programs. By beginning with a pilot project one can develop local expertise and generate enthusiasm amongst learners and teachers. Formative assessments that focus on learning will require fewer resources and demand less stringency regarding case portrayal and rating accuracy than high stakes exams. They are likely to be less stressful for all involved, and thus have a better chance to convert skeptics.

Figure 2.3 shows a worksheet used in planning for our example general internal medicine residency OSCE to assign tasks and prepare a project timeline (a blank copy of this worksheet is also included as Appendix C). Typically one needs to start work 3–4 months before the event. However, with the help of individuals who already have much expertise in this area, shorter planning times may be possible.

Best Practices: OSCE Planning

- Identify date and time of OSCE.
- Make a timeline working backward from the OSCE date.
- Start early to identify potential SPs and secure training times.
- Identify potential location of OSCE early (clinic rooms, class rooms, or simulation center).
- Secure participants' availability.

Fig. 2.1 Example worksheet for making initial OSCE plans

OSCE Project Name	Annual General Internal Medicine Residency OSCE

OSCE Goals	Assessment of general clinical competencies

Number and Type of Trainees	24 PGY-1s

Number and Type of Stations	10 independent stations with SP encounters

Potential Timing	All residents on one Saturday (two 3.5-hour sessions)

Potential Space	Outpatient department when no patient care sessions

Budget Available and Potential Funding Sources	$4,000 + $1,000 possible institutional grant

Motivational Strategies	Snacks for residents and SPs. Two rest stations per resident rotation. Immediate post-station feedback with faculty observers.

Budget Items to Consider	$ Needed	In Kind	Cost per Learner
Space 1 room per station, SP/faculty and learner meeting areas		Donated	
SPs – training & OSCE performance Check for local rates, costs vary depending on location and simulation task. Ask SPs to arrive ½ hour prior to the start of the OSCE and factor early arrival into payment.	4 hrs training + 2 4-hr OSCEs @ $25/hr x 10 cases (+ 2 trained <u>alternates</u>) **$3,200**		**$133.33**
Raters – training & rater tasks I.e., when faculty raters are used instead of or in addition to SPs; consider credit for "teaching" if direct reimbursement of faculty is not possible		Donated	
Refreshments Need not be fancy but can help create a more relaxed atmosphere	$120		$5
Medical Supply Need not be sterile but should be authentic		Donated	
Office Supply Photocopying forms, pens		Donated	
Video Equipment & Supply Sample learner performance for quality control and future learning activities. Cameras may be purchased (a recommended one-time investment!), rented or borrowed.	4 digital cameras @ $200/each + blank DVDs **$840**		**$35**
Data Entry & Report Card Assembly May be performed by in-house or temporary staff	<u>40 hrs @ $15/hr</u> **$600**		**$25**
Data Analysis Faculty/staff with statistical capabilities are vital to an OSCE organization team		Donated*	
TOTAL	**$4,760**		**$198.33**

* If faculty not available, additional cost to hire an outside master's level statistician estimated at $40/hr x 10 hrs = $400

Fig. 2.2 Example OSCE budget. This figure continues the example ten-station General Internal Medicine Residency OSCE outlined in Fig. 2.1. SP training time includes both rater and case portrayal training. Cost per learner is calculated for 24 residents

OSCE Project Name:	Date:
Annual General Internal Medicine Residency OSCE	**March 19th**

	Tasks	Individuals Involved	Deadline
Overall Initial Planning			
3-4 months before the OSCE	▪ Decide on format (e.g., number of stations, time frame)	L, P, SD	Nov. 24th
	▪ Create a blueprint (identify competencies to be assessed)	L, P, SD	Nov. 24th
	▪ Decide on what to maintain from previous OSCEs/develop new cases	L, P	Jan. 1st
	▪ Identify appropriate OSCE location (stations and assembly rooms)	L, P	Dec. 3rd
	▪ Recruit staff (for administrative tasks, monitoring, time keeping)	P	Dec. 17th
	▪ Decide on SP/rater recruitment and training schedule	P	Dec. 17th
	▪ Communicate with learners (e.g., provide dates/times, explain procedure)	L, P	Jan. 7th
	▪ Clarify budget (e.g., SP costs, refreshments)	P	Dec. 17th
	▪ Consider videotaping	L, P	Dec. 17th
Station/Material Preparations			
1 week - 3 months before the OSCE	▪ Review old station/OSCE materials (e.g., learner/SP instructions, rating forms)	L, P, SD, A	Jan. 14th
	▪ Develop new station/OSCE materials (i.e., content generation and formatting)	L, P, SD, A	Jan. 31st
	▪ Determine SP payment process	P, A	Dec. 17th
	▪ Make room arrangements	A	Dec. 17th
	▪ Recruit SPs	P	Feb. 18th
	▪ Train SPs	*!	Mar. 11th
	▪ Recruit faculty	L, P	Jan. 14th
	▪ Prepare faculty (e.g., circulate station/format information, rater training)	P	Feb. 18th
	▪ Prepare props (e.g., fake pill bottles and charts)	P	Mar. 4th

Fig. 2.3 Example worksheet for assigning OSCE responsibilities and creating timelines. "Individuals Involved" follow the OSCE staffing roles listed in Table 2.1 (*L* leader, *P* planner, *A* administrator, *SD* station developer, *Tr* SP trainer, *Ti* timer, *M* monitor, *DM* data manager, *DA* data analyst)

General Preparations

1-2 weeks before the OSCE	▪ Order supplies (e.g., paper, folders)	A	Mar. 4th
	▪ Order refreshments	A	Mar. 14th
	▪ Photocopy station materials	A	Mar. 11th
	▪ Assign SPs, faculty and learners (create assignment sheets)	A	Mar. 4th
	▪ Prepare name tags/labels for learners (assign learner IDs)	A	Mar. 11th
	▪ Develop rotation schedules	A	Mar. 4th
	▪ Prepare invoices and necessary paperwork for SP payment	A	Mar. 4th
	▪ Prepare signs (e.g., station numbers, arrows to signal flow)	A	Mar. 18th
	▪ Orient hall monitors and time keepers	P	Mar. 18th

OSCE Administration

day of the OSCE	▪ Prepare stations and assembly rooms (signs, station materials, refreshments)	M	Mar. 19th
	▪ Assign substitutes (if necessary)	M	Mar. 19th
	▪ Orient faculty, SPs and other personnel	P	Mar. 19th
	▪ Position faculty, SPs, hall monitors and time keepers	M	Mar. 19th
	▪ Orient learners (e.g., assign starting station, disseminate name/number labels)	L	Mar. 19th
	▪ Guide learners to individual starting stations	M	Mar. 19th
	▪ Time stations (start, feedback, station changes)	Ti	Mar. 19th
	▪ Manage emergencies (e.g., equipment breakdown)	M	Mar. 19th
	▪ Assure smooth changeovers of SPs, faculty and learners	M	Mar. 19th
	▪ Reassemble learner group (e.g., for debriefing, program evaluations)	L	Mar. 19th
	▪ Collect and count all forms	A	Mar. 19th
	▪ Clean up stations and assembly rooms	M	Mar. 19th

Post-OSCE Tasks

days to months after the OSCE	▪ Sort out forms	DM	Mar. 21st
	▪ Ensure timely SP payment	A	Mar. 25th
	▪ Enter data and evaluation results	DM	Mar. 25th
	▪ Analyze data	DA	Apr. 8th
	▪ Report evaluation data (e.g., report cards)	P, L	Apr. 19th
	▪ Report on experience internally and externally (e.g., presentations, articles)	L, PE	Sept. 19th

Fig. 2.3 (continued)

Step 3

Establish a Blueprint

A key element for designing an OSCE is the development of a blueprint. This is a matrix that connects a list and brief description of all stations with the competencies that are being assessed (see, e.g., Fig. 2.4; a blank blueprint is included as Appendix D). This ensures that individual competencies are examined multiple times and that each station contributes to the overall comprehensiveness of the exam or exercise by assessing multiple competencies. We create our blueprints by selecting cases from our case bank (see Fig. 2.10), a useful repository which organizes our accumulating cases by key blueprinting information, tracks case usage, and enables tailored querying (e.g., distribution by age, percentage New, Ongoing, Follow-up, and Discharge cases).

An organized approach to blueprinting strengthens an OSCE's validity. This can include literature reviews, curriculum surveys, and consensus building discussions. OSCEs should provide a good cross section of medical encounters typically experienced by learners. If the OSCE is a formative exercise, post-OSCE feedback from trainees (see Appendix K for a participant post-OSCE survey) should confirm that the stations assessed issues they encounter in their current work or are likely to encounter in their future practice.

The final station sequencing is guided by several considerations, including variability of case gender and emotional tone (e.g., two "angry patient" stations should not be next to

Table 2.2 Questions important for blueprint development

- Are cases representative of typical clinical practice?
- Are cases representative of what has been taught in the course/ rotation?
- Do the cases adequately cover all the competencies to be tested?
- Are diagnostic and management challenges varied in a systematic fashion?
- Is there a balance in terms of gender, either equally divided or resembling real life practice?
- Is there an appropriate mix of patient ages?
- Is there an appropriate mix of races and cultural backgrounds?

each other) as well as site or station limitations (e.g., only certain rooms have an external phone connection).

Once a first draft of a blueprint is completed, organizers should ask themselves the questions listed in Table 2.2.

Best Practices: Blueprinting

- Delineate core competencies.
- Establish performance criteria for each level of training.
- Ensure OSCE case patient age, gender, race, and prevalence of disease reflect actual clinical practice.
- Align OSCE skills and content assessed with current or new curricula.

	Station		Skills Assessed				Comments
	Case	Content Areas	Comm	History Gathering	Physical Exam	Treatment Mgmt & Plan	
1	<u>Urethritis Follow-up</u> - take sexual Hx from bisexual pt	Prevention (HIV, sexual Hx, STI prevention)	X	X		X	M. Unlink from lab tests.
2	<u>High Risk Smoker</u> - move pt from contemplation to action stage, develop plan	Addiction Medicine (smoking, behavior change cycle)	X	X		X	M. Adjust case for local pt population.
3	<u>Street Fair</u> - counsel pt about positive bone density results	Geriatrics (osteoporosis, bone density, Dexa interpretation)	X	X		X	F. Clarify instructions, change to Dexa results.
4	<u>Diabetes (phone)</u> - triage problem over the phone	Common Symptoms/ Undifferentiated Problems (DDx of diarrhea), Phone Medicine	X	X		X	F. Adapt case from other program.
5	<u>Difficulty Sleeping</u> - screen appropriately	Common Symptoms/ Undifferentiated Problems (PTSD, DDx of sleep problems)	X	X		X	M/F. Develop new case.
6	<u>Loss of Loved One</u> - counsel pt who recently lost spouse	Common Symptoms/ Undifferentiated Problems (stages of grief, grief counseling)	X			X	F. Emphasize common symptoms or acute problems?
7	<u>Diabetes Precepting</u> - precept SL, new onset diabetes case	Acute Problems (diabetes), Microskills Teaching		X		X	M/F.
8	<u>Asthma</u> - assess tightness in chest, counsel re: medication	Acute Problems (asthma Dx and Tx)	X	X	X	X	F. How many residents got prednisone training?
9	<u>Test Results (phone)</u> - liver abnormalities	Acute Problems, Lab Tests, Phone Medicine	X	X		X	M. Check new recommendations.
10	<u>Teaching Px Skills</u> - teach student Px procedures	Px Procedures, Bedside Teaching (incorporating pt)	X		X		Similar to last year except for procedure.

Fig. 2.4 Example blueprint for an Internal Medicine residency OSCE (*Hx* history, *Px* physical exam, *Dx* diagnosis, *DDx* differential diagnosis, *Tx* treatment, *STI* sexually transmitted infection, *PTSD* posttraumatic stress disorder, *SL* standardized learner)

Step 4

Develop Cases and Stations

A blueprint leads to a profile for each of the stations which then can serve as a starting point for case development (the *case* is the clinical problem; the *station* involves a specific set of tasks being assessed in the OSCE). Basing OSCE stations on real patient cases will add validity. However, after disguising the identity of the source patient, it may be necessary to make adjustments for the training level, OSCE focus, or the time limitations imposed by the exercise. Figure 2.5 illustrates how one can adjust the difficulty level of communication tasks. By making stations more or less challenging one can also increase or decrease the overall difficulty of the OSCE.

Educators should not feel obligated to start from scratch in developing their OSCE cases. Our case development worksheet is included in Appendix I. (Our template follows Silverman et al.'s (2005) History of Present Illness framework and was refined with reference to the Wayne State School of Medicine Standardize Patient Program's (2011)

case development tool.) See also Appendix J for a checklist development worksheet. Additional selected station/case development resources are included in Appendix P (Other Resources). We also recommend reaching out to other health professions schools; many programs will likely be willing to share their OSCE cases.

As part of the station development process it is important to try out new cases through role-play and adherence to the given time limits. Sometimes multiple enactments are necessary to gain clarity on issues such as scope of task or SP emotional tone. Role-play at this stage should involve faculty who know the target learner group and the sort of questions they are likely to ask the SPs.

Case materials for the SP and faculty need to be sufficiently detailed to assure consistency. Yet, they must not be so voluminous that there are too many details to remember and to reproduce consistently. Table 2.3 provides considerations specific to each component of the documentation accompanying each case. A sample case (including station overview, directions for the OSCE participant, and detailed SP case portrayal instructions) plus corresponding rating forms for both the SP and faculty observer are provided in Appendices F, G, and H.

	Less Challenging	**More Challenging**
Data Gathering	<ul><li>history of present illness</li><li>past medical history</li><li>psychosocial history</li><li>occupational/environmental history</li></ul>	<ul><li>sexual history</li><li>substance abuse history</li><li>suicidal ideation</li><li>domestic violence</li><li>cultural/religious practices</li><li>mental status exam</li></ul>
Patient Education & Counseling	<ul><li>simple issues</li><li>aligned health beliefs</li><li>motivated patient</li></ul>	<ul><li>multifaceted problems</li><li>nonaligned health beliefs</li><li>resistant patient</li></ul>
Negotiations & Shared Decision Making	<ul><li>agreement between parties</li><li>understanding</li></ul>	<ul><li>disagreement between parties</li><li>lack of understanding</li></ul>

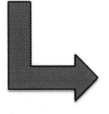

Communication Barriers

- language
- literacy/health literacy
- cultural differences (e.g., dress code)
- altered cognitive state (e.g., intoxication, dementia, confusion)
- intense emotional state (e.g., depression, anger, mania, anxiety, shock, shame)
- difficulty/inability to speak/hear/see
- physical setting (e.g., patient in bed, connected to hospital equipment)
- telephone/online communications
- multiple interviewees/interviewers

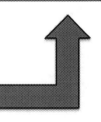

Fig. 2.5 Adjusting a case for station difficulty

Table 2.3 Overview of station-specific materials (their purpose, content, and special considerations)

Forms	Purpose	Content elements	Considerations/tips
Station overview	To assist program organizers	■ Station goals/objectives (what is the purpose of this station) ■ Competencies to be assessed ■ Logistics (personnel, station materials, room arrangements)	■ Be specific ■ Identify room requirements (e.g., telephone access)
Learner instructions	To communicate the scenario and tasks to learners before they enter the station	■ Patient information (e.g., name, age, occupation) ■ Reason for visit ■ Learner role ■ Starting point for encounter (beginning, middle, end) ■ Situation (medical/psychosocial information available, prior developments/encounters) ■ Learner task(s)	■ Be brief (consider reading time) ■ Assure equal length with other stations ■ Timeline with arrows can help orient learner quickly ■ Bulleted information can be read faster ■ Use language learners are familiar with (e.g., well-known abbreviations)
Fact sheets (only in selected stations or OSCEs)	To provide learners with information needed for managing the case if specific information is not familiar or if one tries to focus encounter on communication skills and wants to equalize the required medical knowledge	■ Guidelines for diagnosis and treatment (case specific) ■ Case-specific screening tools (if they would be present in a clinical setting) ■ Administrative or legal factors relevant to the case ■ Community resources	■ Be brief (reading time is limited) ■ Assure parity with other stations ■ Organize material to be reviewed quickly ■ Use graphs where possible ■ Assure accuracy ■ Avoid controversy
SP instructions	To prepare SPs for their case	■ Scenario (what happened from the SPs perspective, why is he/she here today, prior medical encounters) ■ Current life situation and past history (medical and psychosocial) ■ Personality and emotional tone (how to relate to the learner) ■ Cues for learner (verbal, nonverbal) ■ Timing (beginning, middle, end/after 2-min warning)	■ Provide opportunity for SPs to personalize scenario within limits (e.g., name of spouse) ■ Supply an "opening line" and specific messages to give ■ Be specific ■ Balance level of detail (i.e., not too little and not too much) ■ Illustrate the emotional tone to be portrayed with sample statements ■ Clearly identify challenges for the learner/station goals
Rating form	To capture the performance assessments	■ Administrative information (e.g., learner IDs, date, station) ■ Dimensions on which to assess the learner (e.g., communication skills, case management) ■ Checklist or global rating items ■ Room for comments (e.g., areas of strengths, areas in need for improvement)	■ Make items evidence based ■ Keep the number of items manageable for the allotted rating time and for the ability of average raters to focus on during the encounter ■ Watch out for double negatives ■ Pretest for readability and ability to observe and rate ■ Include at least one summary rating for cross-validation
Faculty instructions	To standardize faculty assessment and teaching	■ Procedural steps for observing encounters (e.g., positioning to observe nonverbal behavior, start/stop video) ■ Procedural steps for providing feedback (e.g., start with learner's self-assessment, invite SP to comment) ■ Teaching points (i.e., what messages to deliver to each learner if instant feedback is provided)	■ Keep it brief ■ Use bullets when possible ■ Assure that procedures are consistent at all stations ■ Assure that teaching points match the station goals
Post-encounter materials (optional)	To give learners the opportunity to reflect on/synthesize the encounter, receive feedback, or extend their clinical reasoning about the case	■ Patient note (with space for summarizing history, diagnosis, and treatment plan) ■ Supplementary diagnostic test results (e.g., EKG, X-ray)	■ Be selective and pragmatic: e.g., weigh faculty availability for giving feedback versus gathering further learner data ■ Consider computer- versus paper-based ■ Consider reserving the time between stations for rest with no post-encounter activities

Table 2.4 Guidelines for giving brief instant feedback during the OSCE

1. *Start by asking the learner, "How did it go?"*
2. *Reflect back key points*
3. *Ask SP(s) for feedback (if appropriate)*
4. *Ask the learner what was done well*
   - Be prepared to discuss 1 item from the rating form
   - Must be a specific behavior
5. *Ask the learner what could be done differently*
   - Be prepared to discuss 1 item from the rating form
   - Must be specific behavior
6. *Feed forward*: "The next time you see a patient like this, what will you do?"

Table 2.5 Review questions important for case development or adaptation

- *Are the station goals clear?* Do they provide precise information about what the station is supposed to teach or assess in terms of what learners need to know and what learners need to be able to do?
- *Is the case appropriate for the learner?* Consider profession, training level, course/rotation content
- *Can the tasks be managed or at least initiated in the given time?* (e.g., 10 min)
- *Are the learner instructions clear?* Can someone quickly ascertain what the situation is and what needs to be done? Are the instructions uniform across cases in terms of format and length?
- *Are the SP instructions clear?* Do they provide adequate background information for an SP to take on the role? Do they clearly indicate the key elements of the case, what is essential in terms of content, emotional tone, and timing?
- *Are the faculty instructions clear?* Do they provide adequate guidelines on how the faculty is supposed to proceed? Do they include appropriate, station-specific teaching points if post-encounter feedback is involved?
- *Is it possible to simulate the physical and/or psychological signs and symptoms for the length of time allocated to each rotation?*
  For example, can someone stay who depressed for 10 min? Will the case require multiple SPs because it is too stressful or too difficult to maintain a particular physical finding?
- *Will it be possible to find an adequate number of SPs to portray this case?* If not, can age, gender, or other characteristics be changed to make the search easier?

Each OSCE form should be clearly marked with station number and title. The title needs to be phrased in a way not to give away the sometimes hidden, station-specific challenge (e.g., "Secret Drinker"). In designing a scenario one should also consider how to use the time immediately following the SP encounter. Post-encounter options for the learner include writing up a patient note, interpreting additional diagnostic information, receiving immediate feedback, or, simply, rest. Which option one selects will depend on one's goal for the OSCE and the station, as well as pragmatic considerations

such as faculty availability to observe and debrief encounters (see Table 2.3). If learners receive feedback after each encounter there are typically strict time limits. Thus it is very important to provide clear guidelines for the observer, whether it is a faculty member or the SP. Table 2.4 provides a sample set of instructions that could help structure a brief feedback session. It will also be important to add 2–4 station-specific teaching points to make sure that the teaching objectives for each station are accomplished with each learner. Also see the feedback training protocol (Table 2.11).

To assure the quality of each case, organizers should ask themselves the questions listed in Table 2.5.

Best Practices: Case Development

- Choose scenarios that are both common and challenging presentations for your learners.
- Ensure that cases represent the patient population in your clinical environment.
- Build specific goals and challenges into each scenario.
- Choose a post-encounter activity (i.e., feedback, supplementary exercise, or rest).
- Make sure it is possible to complete tasks in the time allotted.
- Organize a trial run with a variety of other learners to validate and fine tune cases.

Step 5

Create Rating Forms

The quality of a rating form is judged by the degree to which raters, both SPs and/or faculty, can use the form consistently (i.e., reliability, the degree to which the form would produce the same results if used by different raters or on different occasions) and the degree to which the elements of the rating form accurately reflect the intended skills and performance (i.e., validity). The keys to developing reliable and valid rating form items are (a) identifying the specific domains, (b) writing understandable items, and (c) providing anchors or instructions that guide raters in their assessment. By establishing a blueprint which specifies what skills and content the OSCE is designed to assess, and how each station contributes towards this goal, much of the work in creating effective rating forms is already done. The items in the rating form should reflect the blueprint and can therefore include both skills assessed across all stations within an OSCE as well as content and skills specific to a station or subset of stations. Two formats for the rating form items are typically used: behavior-specific items (did the trainee perform a specific behavior?) and global ratings. Both are important (Norcini et al. 2011) and many rating forms include both. These two types of items are usually strongly correlated; however, each may provide unique information about trainee performance. From the perspective of feedback on performance, behavior-specific checklist items provide learners with actionable data while global ratings are much less directive. Space for comments is also useful to provide opportunities to indicate rating challenges or more specifics about the learner's performance (Kachur et al. 1990). Sample rating forms can be found in Appendices G, H, and O. Appendix J provides a checklist development template.

Behavior-Specific Rating Form Items

Table 2.6 provides a stepwise process for developing behavior-specific rating form items. The number of behaviorally anchored items that are assessed within a particular domain affects the quality of the measurement. The more items, the more reliable and valid a rating form is likely to be. The trade-off is the burden on the rater. Asking raters to rate too many and/or very complex aspects of performance can lead to decreased accuracy. Extensive, targeted training of raters and providing adequate time to rate are two additional ways of achieving a good balance.

Checklists are popular in OSCEs because of their simplicity—noting simply whether or not specific behaviors or actions were performed can enhance the accuracy and reliability of ratings. However, such simplification may miss important dimensions of performance and could, in some circumstances, compromise the validity of the assessment tool. In addition, many raters object to simple yes/no checklists because so much of the behavior they witness falls into an area between those dichotomies. Thus scales that provide multiple rating options (e.g., Likert-type or forced choice formats) are

Table 2.6 Stepwise process for creating behavior-specific rating form items

1. *Conceptualize the competencies needed to perform the station task well* e.g., communication skills, physical exam skills
2. *Compare that conceptualization with available standards* e.g., literature, experts
3. *Operationalize the competencies to turn them into written items* e.g., uses open-ended questions, asks about alcohol use
4. *Determine the rating options* i.e., done/not done checklist versus scale
5. *Create behavioral anchors to help evaluators identify which rating option to select* e.g., if done more than once
6. *Pilot the rating form* multiple times if possible
7. *Refine the rating form*

often preferred. While more response options offer raters more opportunities to report on fine nuances, they can also complicate the rater's decision-making process, may take up valuable rating time, and can lead to a reduction in reliability if the response options don't align well with learner behavior.

One compromise is to use a trichotomous anchoring system, such as "not done," "partly done," "well done." This approach seems to help overcome the tendency of many raters to "give credit" to learners whenever possible and also helps set a high standard for performance. Looking ahead at the interpretation of performance data which will result from the OSCE, one can then create summary scores that represent the proportion or percent of items rated as "done well" versus "partly or not done." When identifying appropriate behavioral anchors for each of these response options, it is important to consider the level of the learner and the likely distribution of competence in the learner population in order to avoid floor (everyone does poorly) and ceiling (everyone does well) effects and maximize the degree to which the items differentiate among learners.

Global Rating Form Items

Global ratings address general impressions about a learner's performance in a particular domain (e.g., communication skills, medical knowledge, professionalism) or they may also address overall satisfaction with an encounter. SPs are often asked to indicate the degree to which they would recommend the learner as a physician to a family member or friend, reflecting measures widely used with "real" patients to assess patient satisfaction and quality of care.

Global ratings are often thought to be less reliable because they are not anchored in specific, observable behavior and therefore more susceptible to the subjectivity of the rater. However, in certain situations—with "expert" raters evaluating more holistic competence—global ratings may be more valid than checklist ratings.

Such broad assessments provide an overall "gestalt," and include more intuitive aspects of the raters' judgments. They may even capture performance elements that are not reflected in the behavioral-specific items. Generally the reliability of global ratings has been quite satisfactory (Hodges & McIlroy 2003). Often such ratings use a 4- or 5-point scale and have specific anchors. For example, recommendation ratings ("would you recommend this physician to a family member or friend?") can use simple descriptions such as "not recommend," "recommend with reservations," "recommend," "highly recommend," or more specific, complex descriptions of exemplar levels of performance that constitute each point on the scale. Global ratings require less attention to performance details and thus less memorization for SPs. On the other hand, there are many (often uncontrolled) factors that influence them, including subjective biases like halo, availability, social comparison, and selective attention biases. In addition, formative feedback is difficult to provide on the basis of such global ratings.

Best Practices: OSCE Checklists

- Develop rating items based on the blueprint and ensure that a sufficient number of items are included to reliably assess competence within the targeted domains.
- Consider using both behavior-specific items and global rating items in OSCE rating forms to achieve a balance in terms of helping raters reflect important elements of their subjective responses and to enhance their objectivity in representing what happened during the encounter and providing learners with specific and more holistic feedback.
- Develop response options for behavior-specific items that reflect observable actions and strive to match the response options to the likely variation in performance of the learner population to maximize differentiation.

Step 6

Recruit and Train SPs

Recruitment

Think of choosing SPs as a theater director would cast a show. Each case has unique requirements, some are physiological, others are psychological. Before starting with the recruitment process it is helpful to list all physical or psychological characteristics that would jeopardize the succinct portrayal of a case. Physiological contraindications may include scars, atrophied injection sites of insulin-dependent diabetics, respiratory ailments, heart murmurs, or other physical findings may diminish the fidelity of the case. Psychological contraindications may include discomfort in exposing one's body if a physical exam is part of that station, inability to express emotions if pain is of importance in the case, or a hostile interpersonal approach if the case asks for a withholding attitude. Casting the right person for the case is important for creating an appropriate degree of realism. Even when they are experienced actors, it is difficult for SPs to overcome their typical ways of behaving or expressing themselves. If a person is exceptionally outgoing and actively expressing emotions through nonverbal behavior, then a case where tiredness and lethargy are the issue may be less appropriate. The energy to transfer a very active style into a passive one may distract from other tasks such as remembering the history items or evaluating the trainee.

Table 2.7 SP characteristics that simplify training

SP characteristic		Effect on training
Acting experience	⇨	Less need to train acting (especially of high emotional levels)
Health care professionals (or trainees in the health professions)	⇨	More understanding of learner role and technical issues (e.g., interview, physical exam)
No personal expertise with the case problem	⇨	Less emotional involvement with the case
Personal experience with the case problem	⇨	Disease-related knowledge is already present
Type casted	⇨	Less need to teach affect
Prior SP experience	⇨	Less need to teach the mechanics of OSCEs
Use of SPs own background	⇨	Less history information to remember
Over age 18	⇨	No need for developmental considerations
Under age 70	⇨	Easier to train, may remember better
GTA or UTA experience	⇨	Comfortable with physical exams, used to focus on performance details, expert in breast and pelvic or urological exams

GTA gynecological teaching associate, *UTA* urology teaching associate

Familiarity with the medical problem in focus can either help or hinder the simulation. On one hand, having experienced a medical problem oneself may provide special insights into the case. On the other hand, memories about own interactions with health care professionals may overshadow the encounter with the learner and may provide a hazard to standardization of the case portrayal or to rater tasks. To avoid an increased need for SP maintenance, it is better to select SPs for whom the medical problem in focus does not evoke special memories. As Table 2.7 illustrates, by looking ahead at training requirements one can consider some SP characteristics that are likely to reduce the need for preparations.

In general, SPs must be able to control their emotions well. For example, they cannot appear upset if something tragic happened in their real life and cannot explode on the examinees because they are angry with the project administration. This type of job takes someone who does not burst into laughter if a trainee reacts in an unusual fashion, asks strange questions, or even attempts to make the SP break role. SPs also need to be comfortable in cross-cultural encounters since learners may be from many different backgrounds.

Actors have been viewed by many as ideal candidates. Professionals or amateurs, these are people who like to slip in and out of roles and may jump at an opportunity to do so. However, it will be important to clarify for them that working as SP is not a creative act. Even though much improvisation is needed, the focus is on standardization. Not every actor is willing to go along with that, and often times a real acting opportunity will be preferable to taking on an "educational" role. Thus the OSCE project can quickly be missing an SP.

Once a program has developed a cadre of SPs, word of mouth will often become the most effective and efficient way of recruitment. One experienced SP coordinator felt that a referral from another SP has a one in two chance of bringing in a good candidate, with a physician referral the chances are one in three. Using ads, only 1 in 20 responses may lead to hiring (Tamblyn et al. 1991).

Training for Case Portrayal

To make a patient's case come to life SPs need to become accomplished in three different areas. (1) They must know all the physical, psychological, and social details related to their case. (2) They must be able to consistently portray the right emotional tone—not too much and not too little, but just the right amount that fits the case. (3) Their actions and responses must be timed correctly. Many novice SPs tend to give away all the information they have about the case right up front, maybe even feeling some relief to have gotten the story right. However, often we want learners to practice or demonstrate skills for eliciting information and thus, sharing information prematurely reduces the learner's chances to

work on important skills. Since OSCE encounters are time limited, it is important that learners have a chance to come to some closure. A continuation of questioning or emotional intensity could make that impossible. Thus SPs need to learn to pace themselves and to adhere to warning knocks or other indicators that the encounter needs to come to an end.

Whenever more than one SP is to be prepared for the same case, group training is necessary for standardization. SPs can read through the case together while clarifications are provided. They can even view a standard setting videotape to emphasize nonverbal behavior and emotional tone. Role-playing the case multiple times with trainers as well as each other is essential. It is also helpful to expose SPs to good as well as poor learner performances. By practicing with each other, SPs can gain important insights into the interviewer role and gain empathy for learners.

Table 2.8 lays out a protocol for training SPs. For logistical reasons or time limitations it may not always be possible to go through all steps, but one could consider those in the shaded boxes as the most essential ones. There are varied opinions as to how much training is necessary for SPs to perform their case adequately. A relevant book on SP training advocates a 5-session approach: (1) Familiarization with the Case; (2) Learning to Use the Checklist; (3) Putting it All Together (Performance, Checklist, Feedback); (4) first Dress Rehearsal; (5) Final Dress Rehearsal (Wallace 2007). The total amount of training time will depend on case requirements,

Table 2.8 Training protocol: SP portrayal

1. *Provide training program overview* e.g., when and how to get where, who will they be working with, what are the program objectives, what is the history of the project, what will a typical encounter with learners be like, who else will be in the room, what prior experience learners will have had with OSCEs/SPs

2. *Explore SP expectations/concerns* e.g., prior work with learners at the targeted training level—how did it go, how did it compare to their expectations, what are their concerns, what are they looking forward to, how might it be similar/different from previous SP work

3. *Review individual cases* break into subgroups, have SPs take turns reading aloud the learner instructions, SP instructions, and rating form, stop along the way to explain, elicit emotional reactions, jointly come up with additional information to round out the case (e.g., name of spouse, home address), clarify:
   - Case content, story, what information needs to be conveyed
   - Emotional tone, type, and intensity
   - Timing of SP interventions, what to say/do in the beginning, middle, end of the encounter or only upon prompting by the learner

4. *Review video sample encounter* to get at emotional tone, nonverbal behavior, bring out more of SPs past simulation experiences, show learner's expected level of performance

5. *Demonstrate SP encounters* select SP volunteer or SP who has portrayed same or similar case before, others watch while referring to SP instructions and rating forms, time the encounter as you would during the OSCE, model what would happen during and after the encounter (e.g., physical exam, rating, feedback), discuss case portrayal, recheck the SP instructions if indicated, if there are multiple demonstration interviews change SPs and modify interviewer approach (e.g., poor performance, unprofessional behavior)

6. *Videotape practice encounters and review performance* reviews can be done in a group or SPs can watch tapes independently and then discuss their impressions and reactions

7. *SPs practice with each other* make sure everyone takes on the learner role at least once to appreciate the challenges involved in the case, reduce anxiety performance by "requesting" the interviewing SP to make mistakes as a learner might, include rating and feedback to learner in role-play (if applicable)

8. *Organize trial runs* the more practice, the more SPs will learn about potential learner approaches to the case (e.g., questions, physical exam maneuvers), organizing a mock OSCE (if possible in the place where the real OSCE will occur) can provide unique practice opportunities and greatly enhance understanding of context and timing

cost, and time limitations. If it is a formative assessment 2 h may be adequate, especially with SPs who have experience. If it is a summative assessment, training will have to be much more extensive and, there are literature reports of 10–20 h of training (ibid). However, the latter will have to be divided into shorter training segments. Typically 2 h is a limit to how much SPs can absorb at one time. We typically train SPs for 4–6 h, including a minimum of 2 h focusing on the case and 2 h on the checklist. When organizing a higher-stakes event one must definitely consider a trial run. New SPs can especially benefit from getting a first-hand experience of the tasks and timing involved.

Best Practices: SP Recruitment and Training

- Search for SPs through word-of-mouth strategies (e.g., by contacting other SPs, connecting with other SP trainers, talking to clinicians and acting teachers).
- Cast the right person for each case (i.e., physical appearance, psychological profile, availability, no contraindications).
- For high stakes programs recruit and train alternates who can step in if needed (alternates can be cross-trained to provide coverage for multiple cases).
- Put SPs into learner's positions through role-play to enhance their understanding of the case (e.g., interactive and emotional impact of SP actions) and to promote an empathic approach to learners.
- Practice all aspects of the encounter (e.g., physical exam, feedback); do not leave SP performance to chance.
- Explore the psychological and physiological impact a case has on the SP to avoid toxic side effects (e.g., getting depressed from repeatedly portraying a depressed patient, getting muscle spasms from portraying a patient who has difficulty walking).
- Train all SPs who are portraying the same case (simultaneously or consecutively) at the same time to enhance consistency in case portrayal across SPs.

Step 7

Recruit and Train Evaluators

An important decision when planning an OSCE is who will rate the participants. Depending on the OSCE project, faculty, SPs, and/or peers will be entrusted with the responsibility of rating a trainee's performance. At times evaluations are completed by more than one group of observers. Often organizers do not have the luxury to select raters even though some research suggests that recruiting the right people might be more important than training them (Newble et al. 1980). An initial rater screening strategy could consist of assembling candidates in small groups and showing them selected videotapes of station encounters. By setting a required level of inter-rater and test–retest reliability one can quantify the suitability and readiness of the candidates in question. In projects where major promotion decisions depend on OSCE performance, one may even go as far as certifying observers. On the surface, faculty raters may appear ideal, but they are not necessarily accurate (Kalet et al. 1992) and often have limited availability. Many programs use SP raters since they can achieve a good level of reliability, offer the "patient" perspective, are more easily trained, and their availability is already established when signing them on for SP work.

Regardless of whether the rating is done by SPs, faculty, or peers, attention must be given to raters providing as accurate and reliable ratings as possible. The rater task is difficult because there are so many factors that can interfere with an accurate performance assessment. Generally there are three elements to rating a learner's performance: (1) observation of specific behaviors (technique and content), (2) judgment of the behavior against a set of standards, and (3) documentation of the rating. Problems can occur at each of these rater tasks as illustrated in the rater self-assessment guide in Table 2.9.

Raters need to be aware of their rating style, whether they are "doves" (i.e., easy raters) or "hawks" (i.e., harsh raters), and what types of errors they are more likely to make. Self-awareness is no guarantee of being completely error free, but it is the best chance to provide a fair rating.

If possible, raters should be trained groups. A rater training protocol is detailed in Table 2.10. The amount of training time will vary significantly depending on who the raters are, how much rating and OSCE experience they already have, how stringent the assessment is and how much time is available. With clinician raters, it may be most difficult to carve out some training time if no compensation can be provided. However, they too, need some type of orientation, if necessary in writing, to orient them to the goals, process, and content of the exercise.

Attitudes and emotions undoubtedly play a central role in the rating process. It is important for trainers to be aware of how raters feel about the project and their task. Since not everybody can be involved in exam development, raters must at least understand the underlying rationale and feel confident that categories were not selected arbitrarily. Rater trainers have to continuously encourage questions. Although questions add to training time, they are better dealt with before the OSCE starts than while it is in progress or, even worse, when the project is over and one realizes that a rating form item has been completely misunderstood.

Table 2.9 Helping raters improve their accuracy (rater self-assessment guide)

	Key question	WHAT I NEED TO WATCH OUT FOR:
Observation	*What knowledge, skills and attitudes did I observe?*	■ *Too little, too much, or selective attention to details* inappropriate focus ■ *Halo effect* one observation which is easy to obtain or of great significance to rater influences perception of other behavior—first impression error ■ *Observation is too short or too long* premature closure or loss of information
	↓	
Judgment	*How should I rate this trainee on this item?*	■ *Gravitation towards the mean or extremes* central tendency/end-aversion bias or overused end scale points result in too little or too much range ■ *Similar-to-me effect* trainees more similar to rater receive better scores ■ *Contrast effect error* trainees are evaluated against each other and not against an external standard ■ *Generalizations, prejudices, and stereotyping* ■ *Standards are not fully understood* unclear about expectations for training levels ■ *Differences between rating scale points are unclear* ■ *Rater style*: __ dove, __ moderate, __ hawk ■ *Mum effect* hesitation to provide poor performance ratings
	↓	
Documentation	*How do I complete the rating form?*	■ *Incorrect recording* evaluation judgment is not properly marked off ■ *Inadequate or missing comments*

Table 2.10 Training protocol: rating

1. *Provide training program overview* e.g., when to get where, who will they be working with, what are the program objectives, what is the history of the project, what will a typical encounter with learners be like, who else will be in the room, what prior experience learners will have had with OSCEs/SPs

2. *Explore rater expectations/concerns* e.g., prior work with learners at the targeted training level—how did it go, how did it compare to their expectations, what are their concerns, what are they looking forward to, how might it be similar/different from previous rater work

3. *Review case to be observed and rated*
   • Provide a copy of the rating form and define each item (providing examples for the response options)
   • Provide all other case materials (including learner and SP instructions)
   • Let the rater take on the role of a learner to get a personal experience of the case challenges

4. *Perform practice ratings*
   • Use live encounters or videos to demonstrate a "gold standard" evaluation to establish intra- and inter-rater reliability
   • Compare ratings within the group until a consensus is reached
   • Help raters pace themselves by using OSCE-specific time frames (if possible, organize trial runs in the place where the OSCE will take place)

5. *Review typical rater errors* discuss factors that can interfere with rating tasks (see self-assessment form in Table 2.8), encourage raters to become aware of their own style and tendencies

6. *Introduce raters and SPs* (if rating is done by a faculty observer)
   • Encourage them to work together without sharing their individual impressions about the learner's performance before documenting their own ratings
   • Give raters and SPs time to be alone to get to know each other before the first learner arrives
   • Request that they play through the case with the rater taking on the learner role to build understanding and empathy

Table 2.11 Training protocol: feedback

1. *Provide a feedback framework*
   - Explain the behavior change model which helps diagnose learners as pre-contemplative, contemplative, ready for action, in maintenance or relapse stage. Using this framework, feedback can be tailored to optimize its impact on learning
   - Share learner feedback about the feedback (i.e., what learners gained from feedback in post-OSCE debriefing sessions or on program evaluation forms)
2. *Introduce characteristics of effective feedback—written or verbal*
   - Learner self-assessment first
   - Specific not general
   - Focus on behaviors that can be changed, not on personality or other unchangeable characteristics
   - Take advantage of all observers in the station
   - Connect station with previous experiences (e.g., have you had a similar case?)
   - Explore what could be done differently next time (feed forward)
3. *Provide feedback anchors* i.e., teaching points specific for the case that should be covered to strengthen the overall message
4. *Practice giving feedback* e.g., utilizing a video of a performance and role-play

Often in many OSCEs, raters are also asked to provide immediate feedback. Typically there are time limitations (5–10 min) and feedback providers need to be brief. Table 2.11 provides a sample protocol that could help structure a brief feedback session. It will also be important to add 2–4 station-specific teaching points to make sure that the teaching objectives for each station are accomplished with each learner. Providing succinct and meaningful feedback is not always that easy. If raters are also expected to give feedback they should practice doing so in advance of the OSCE (Hatchett et al. 2004).

Best Practices: Evaluator Recruitment and Training for Rating and Feedback Tasks

- Select evaluators who are willing to adopt the program values, who are consistent in their ratings and don't have an ax to grind.
- Bring multiple evaluators together to jointly observe a learner performance on tape or live, compare ratings, and discuss similarities and discrepancies. Practice giving feedback (if this is expected).
- Make raters aware of potential biases and rating mistakes.
- Provide written guidelines for rating items, evaluation scheme, and station objectives/teaching points.
- Post-OSCE, give feedback to raters about how their ratings compare with those of others (e.g., more or less lenient, lack of range).

Step 8

Implement the OSCE: Managing the Session

In addition to station-specific materials, it is also necessary to develop forms and other resources that help with the overall organization of the event. Table 2.12 details the various forms that will be needed. Figure 2.6 provides an example station rotation schedule for OSCE participants, and Fig. 2.7 shows the same schedule from the perspective of the SP/rater. The OSCE participant schedule is also included in blank worksheet form in the back of this book (Appendix E) along with program evaluation surveys (Appendices K–M).

Whenever one plans an event that involves a large number of people, organization can be challenging. One must accept the fact that irregularities will occur, but with good planning and adequate resources, one should be able to make the program manageable. To make trouble shooting at the time of the OSCE easier, it is helpful to contemplate potential solutions ahead of the event. Key concerns include attendance, standardization, time and emotion management. Organizers should ask themselves what they could do in the event of the contingencies listed in Table 2.13. We have included some solutions that have worked for us. By having extra SPs and faculty on hand one can overcome lateness or absences. Adequate training, extra props, and forms can help with standardization. Small time and personnel adjustments may be necessary to keep the OSCE on schedule. Organizers and monitors need to be on the lookout for nervous learners who

Table 2.12 General OSCE materials

Forms	Purpose	Content elements	Considerations/tips
Learner orientation materials	To record attendance and assign ID codes (if applicable)	■ OSCE name, location, date ■ Learner names and ID codes	■ Provide consent forms (if appropriate)
SP/rater orientation materials	To record attendance and match SP/rater names with ID codes (if applicable)	■ Location, date, OSCE number ■ SP/rater names and ID codes	■ Permit room for multiple SPs per station if alternates ■ Allow room for comments and to record special occurrences ■ Provide forms for SPs or others to receive payment
Rotation schedules	To guide the flow of the OSCE, indicate what station learners start with and track where they should be at any given time	■ OSCE name, location, date ■ List of participant names/IDs ■ Areas for indicating rotation periods ■ Station sequence ■ Rest stations or general breaks (if applicable)	■ Add time parameters as reminder (e.g., minutes allowed for SP encounter) ■ Allow room for comments and to record special occurrences ■ Provide room for monitor(s) name(s)
Learner post-OSCE program evaluation forms	To evaluate the OSCE	■ Self-assessment of performance ■ Prior exposure to clinical tasks/cases ■ Emotional reaction to stations ■ Realism of stations ■ Representativeness of performance ■ Motivation to perform well	■ Keep it brief ■ Comments can provide interesting qualitative data
SP and faculty program evaluation forms	To evaluate the OSCE	■ Level of case difficulty ■ Educational value ■ Faculty development value (if faculty rating) ■ SP performance (if faculty rating) ■ Level of enjoyment ■ Appropriateness of case ■ Effectiveness of instructions	■ Keep it brief ■ Comments can provide interesting qualitative data

Table 2.13 OSCE troubleshooting: potential problems and possible remedies

What if…

■ *Someone doesn't show?* For high-stakes OSCEs, always cast and train extra SPs. Consider scheduling open slots into the participant exam schedule to accommodate unforeseen emergencies. For formative OSCEs, ask a faculty member to portray the patient

■ *Someone has to leave temporarily?* Participants and SPs should be informed in advance when designated breaks will occur. For long exams it is a good idea to cast and train multiple SPs for individual stations (While this requires more extensive training to standardize performance and rating across SPs, it ensures an "understudy" will always be on hand)

■ *A rater does not complete the forms correctly?* Designate a staff member to regularly review and count all forms during the OSCE so rating errors can be corrected in real time

■ *A participant enters the wrong station?* Make sure exam proctors are monitoring the exam and can make timely substitutions in the trainee rotation schedule

■ *Timing is off-schedule?* If a station goes overtime, try shortening subsequent rotations by small increments until the schedule is back on track

■ *Someone is late or has to leave early?* Again, make sure time expectations are clear, and prepare back-up SPs

■ *An SP does not portray the case correctly?* Schedule ample training so that everyone is happy with the case portrayal before the actual OSCE. Make sure there is a staff member familiar with the cases present at the OSCE to answer any questions of SPs that may arise in student encounters. Consider videotaping OSCE stations for quality-control post-OSCE

■ *Station materials are missing?* Bring extras of everything, including any props and all forms. Determine in advance the easiest way to make emergency paper copies

■ *Some stations consistently take less than the allotted time?* Check in with the SP between rotations; adjust details of the case portrayal if needed (This is not necessarily a problem)

■ *The OSCE is running out of time?* A participant's "score" in an OSCE is based on his or her performance in multiple stations and should not be compromised as a result of exam scheduling delays. Try first to see if SP and participant can stay late to finish the OSCE

Rotation Schedule for: *General Internal Medicine Residency OSCE*
Date: **March 19ᵗʰ (PM Session)**

Station #	Rotation (# & start time)											
	1	**2**	**3**	**4**	**5**	**6**	**7**	**8**	**9**	**10**	**11**	**12**
Participant ↘	1:00	1:18	1:36	1:54	2:12	2:30	2:48	3:06	3:24	3:42	4:00	4:18 *
Dr. A	1	2	3	4	5	rest	6	7	8	9	10	rest
Dr. B	2	3	4	5	rest	6	7	8	9	10	rest	1
Dr. C	3	4	5	rest	6	7	8	9	10	rest	1	2
Dr. D	4	5	rest	6	7	8	9	10	rest	1	2	3
Dr. E	5	rest	6	7	8	9	10	rest	1	2	3	4
Dr. F	rest	6	7	8	9	10	rest	1	2	3	4	5
Dr. G	6	7	8	9	10	rest	1	2	3	4	5	rest
Dr. H	7	8	9	10	rest	1	2	3	4	5	rest	6
Dr. I	8	9	10	rest	1	2	3	4	5	rest	6	7
Dr. J	9	10	rest	1	2	3	4	5	rest	6	7	8
Dr. K	10	rest	1	2	3	4	5	rest	6	7	8	9
Dr. L	rest	1	2	3	4	5	rest	6	7	8	9	10

*Last station ends at 4:36 pm; debriefing with faculty and residents after the last station

Fig. 2.6 Example OSCE participant rotation schedule. Shown here are the order of rotations (including two rest periods) for half of the 24 residents in our example ten-station OSCE. Each 18-min rotation period includes 5 min feedback. Participant ID numbers may be substituted for names where confidentiality is required (e.g., in a higher-stakes OSCE)

Rotation Schedule for: *General Internal Medicine Residency OSCE*
Date: *March 19th (PM Session)*

Participant	Rotation (# & start time)											
	1	2	3	4	5	6	7	8	9	10	11	12
Station ↘	1:00	1:18	1:36	1:54	2:12	2:30	2:48	3:06	3:24	3:42	4:00	4:18
1 – Urethritis follow-up	A	L	K	J	I	H	G	F	E	D	C	B
2 – Smoker	B	A	L	K	J	I	H	G	F	E	D	C
3 – Street fair	C	B	A	L	K	J	I	H	G	F	E	D
4 – Diarrhea (phone)	D	C	B	A	L	K	J	I	H	G	F	E
5 – Difficulty sleeping	E	D	C	B	A	L	K	J	I	H	G	F
6 – Loss of loved one	G	F	E	D	C	B	A	L	K	J	I	H
7 – Diabetes precepting	H	G	F	E	D	C	B	A	L	K	J	I
8 – Asthma	I	H	G	F	E	D	C	B	A	L	K	J
9 – Test results (phone)	J	I	H	G	F	E	D	C	B	A	L	K
10 – Teaching Px skills	K	J	I	H	G	F	E	D	C	B	A	L

Fig. 2.7 Example OSCE SP/rater rotation schedule. This figure presents the same schedule as in Fig. 2.6, now highlighting the order of residents passing through each station

Best Practices: Optimizing the Test Environment

- Conduct a "dress rehearsal" prior to any high-stakes OSCE.
- Come prepared with extra forms and knowledge of office facilities (computers, printing, copying) near the testing site.
- In designing the OSCE rotation schedule, include time for orientating learners and SPs, as well as time between scenarios and after for post-OSCE debriefing.
- SPs can optimally perform and rate for up to 180 min. There should be a break if you are doing two OSCE sessions on 1 day.
- If the location is not a simulation center then testing staff should include one proctor for each clinical area (e.g., hallway) and one overall administrator.

may enter stations too early or tired SPs who do not portray their case correctly anymore. Post-OSCE debriefing will be useful for all involved.

Step 9

Manage, Analyze, and Report Data

It's important to identify resources and make a plan for entering, managing, and analyzing data early on in the OSCE development process so that you do not end up with poor quality or uninterpretable data—or worse yet, missing data. To do this, "begin with the end in mind" by clarifying what information you hope to obtain from the OSCE and planning accordingly. We have found that good data management practice—which includes protecting trainee privacy—is crucial because it not only ensures high quality data but also helps create a safe learning environment for your trainees. How you handle, use, and report trainee data may be dictated by institutional policy, accreditation regulations, or the law. If you anticipate wanting to conduct research using OSCE data, it is particularly important to understand local policies and regulations with regard to treating trainees as human subjects early in the planning process.

Managing Data

Since it is likely that multiple people will be involved in handling the data from an OSCE, good data management principles should be employed to ensure confidentiality and the integrity and security of the data. Table 2.14 provides a step-by-step approach to addressing privacy concerns.

Ideally, data from OSCEs should be entered directly by raters into user-friendly computer interfaces that then download the data into formats that can be readily uploaded into statistical analysis software (e.g., SPSS, R, SAS) for analysis. If paper rating forms are used, it is good practice to collate data as soon as possible in order to be able to identify any problems with the quality of the data (e.g., inconsistent ratings, missing data, missing learner IDs) and to be able to resolve any problems while memory of the logistics are still fresh (e.g., data are missing because someone arrived late).

While data can be initially entered into a spreadsheet (e.g., Microsoft Excel), which is familiar to most people, we recommend the use of data entry forms that facilitate fast, consistent, and error-free data recording that are easily exported into analyzable formats while ensuring that data fields are accurately labeled. Such forms can be created in "off the shelf" software (e.g., Microsoft Access) or using "open-source" free programs (e.g., Epi Info [wwwn.cdc.gov/epiinfo]; FormSite [www.formsite.com]).

Field-based data entry also facilitates the creation of a "data dictionary" that provides information on each data item (e.g., the checklist item it represents and in which case it was asked), how the response options were entered (e.g., 0=no; 1=yes; or 1–4 for global ratings), the identity of the raters (often good practice to develop an ID system for identifying the SPs), and any issues or problems that should be noted relevant to the OSCE. It's always a good idea to have an OSCE summary sheet that lists important details about each OSCE: date, location, learners, raters, cases, problems, where data is stored and status of data, etc.

Analyzing OSCE Data

Start with descriptive statistics such as distributions of ratings across the response categories (frequencies) for each item on

Table 2.14 Creating a secure and confidential OSCE data storage system

1. *Generate a unique ID for each individual learner* e.g., 4-digit number
2. *In a two-column table, link these new IDs to learners' names and other identifying information* (e.g., email address, schools attended, system IDs)
3. *Store hard and electronic copies of the table in secure locations* e.g., password-protected database file, locked file cabinet; limit access to those with responsibility for learner assessment
4. *Store OSCE data with the unique ID ONLY* i.e., delete all other identifiers
5. *Create a regular system for backing up your data*

the checklist to identify data entry errors and missing data. Then, once you feel the database is accurate, summarize the data across learners to identify program-level gaps in training for specific skills and to establish norms for the group (see Fig. 2.8). Reviewing the data in this detail will help in understanding how to summarize the data for individual learners and for the cohort of learners and will also provide guidance to improve the checklists.

Calculating and Interpreting OSCE Scores

The reasons for calculating OSCE scores are: (1) To set minimum standards for high stakes, pass/fail examinations; (2) To provide feedback to learners (and their faculty) on performance; and (3) To provide overall feedback to your program on the effectiveness of training.

Scores can be based on averages of scaled items or on percentages; the latter are used especially for checklist scores (e.g., percentage of behaviors "done"). If scaled items are non-normally distributed because response options represent a ranking but no clear numerical interpretation, nonparametric statistics can be used (e.g., Cochran's Q, Friedman's Chi Square, Wilcoxon Signed Ranks). For each OSCE, multiple scores can be calculated:

1. Overall OSCE scores: For each station, calculate a summary score (e.g., percentage of maximum points achieved, mean of scaled items). Then average or sum up the station scores across the OSCE. It is best to calculate station scores only when the station was designed to assess a defined skills-set as an overall score (e.g., physical examination, history gathering, communication, etc.). In an OSCE station calling for performance of many skills an overall score can obscure relevant information because it creates one summary score across multiple skill domains.

2. Domain scores: For each station calculate subscores (e.g., percentage of maximum points achieved, mean of scaled items) for the items representing specific domains or categories of skill/performance (e.g., com-munication skills, counseling). Then average or sum up the subscores across all stations where a particular domain was assessed.

When designing a blueprint (Step 3, above) one needs to make sure that each competency/domain is assessed in more than one station. Thus learners have more than one opportunity to demonstrate their skills. As a result, their scores are a more reliable indication of their competence—generally specific skills should be assessed across a minimum of three cases in order to achieve minimum reliability. In most OSCEs, the same core communication skills are assessed in every case because interpersonal and communication skills typically generalize across clinical scenarios. Consequently

most assessments report "communication" performance as a summative (across cases) score.

Assessing the Quality of the OSCE Data

Whenever one organizes an assessment of competence for summative purposes, one needs to be concerned with a variety of psychometric standards, focused mainly on establishing the reliability and validity of the measure. Table 2.15 provides definitions of these key psychometric issues, describes the questions they address, and provides information on strategies for enhancing the quality of the assessment.

When evaluating the quality of your OSCE data, the first question to explore is: To what degree do ratings of learners' performance across the OSCE stations consistently assess learners' underlying competence? This question focuses on inter-station reliability or the internal consistency of the items which assess specific domains across stations and are then used to derive summary OSCE scores. Estimates of internal consistency, or the degree to which sets of assessment items "hang together" (i.e., that a learner who does well on such items in one case will do well on those items in another case) can be calculated using Cronbach's alpha (available in most statistical software programs). Calculating Cronbach's alpha can also identify problematic items—items that were not used consistently by SPs, that were worded in ways that interfered with interpretations, or that do not end up reflecting performance in a particular station—and deleting these items may improve the overall internal consistency of items compromising a summary OSCE score. In most statistical software programs, output for Cronbach's alpha can include what the alpha would be for each set of items if that item were deleted, showing whether individual items enhance or attenuate overall reliability. Cronbach's alphas range from 0 to 1 and generally estimates above 0.80 suggest that items are internally consistent. For pilot OSCEs and OSCEs with fewer stations, Cronbach's alphas should probably exceed 0.60 or 0.70. The consistency of the checklist can also be assessed by estimating test–retest reliability (comparing performance scores for trainees who complete the same OSCE or case without intervening training or education) and inter- or intra-rater reliability (comparing checklist ratings among different raters or over time within the same rater).

Once the reliability of a checklist has been established, attention should turn to gathering evidence of its validity, that is, the degree to which it measures what it was intended to measure. There is no simple way to establish validity and instead efforts to support the validity of a checklist should be based on how well it performs: Does it discriminate among trainees at different levels? Is performance in the OSCE, as measured by the checklists, significantly associated with other measures of related skills (e.g., patient satisfaction, faculty

Student Number (Attach label here)

Evaluator's Name: _____

You have 10 minutes to complete this checklist

OSCE CHECKLIST

COMMUNICATION SKILLS	Not Done	Partly Done	Well Done
Opening			
Introduced self	Did not introduce self **0.7%**	Introduced self only by name and student status **62.4%**	Gave name, student status, and purpose of interview **36.9%**
Information Gathering			
Started with **open-ended** questions	Started with closed, yes/no questions **1.4%**	Began with open-ended questions but stopped prematurely **24.1%**	Started with open-ended questions and continued using them as appropriate **74.5%**
Asked you **what you thought** was the matter	Did not specifically ask **67.8%**	Asked but did not give you enough time to share views **12.1%**	Asked so that you fully shared your views **20.1%**
Managed the **narrative flow** of your story.	Not able to elicit your story because questions not organized logically **6.8%**	Elicited main elements of story, but illogical order of questions disrupted flow **31.1%**	Elicited full story by asking questions that facilitated natural flow of story **62.2%**
Elicited your story using **appropriate questions.**	Impeded story by asking leading questions or more than one question at a time **7.5%**	Used some leading questions and/or asked more than one question at a time, but still able to share most of story **50.0%**	Facilitated the telling of your story by asking questions one at a time without leading you in your responses **42.5%**
Clarified information by repeating to make sure he/she understood you on an ongoing basis	Did not clarify (did not repeat info you provided) **20.1%**	Repeated the information but didn't give you chance to indicate whether accurate **24.8%**	Repeated information and directly invited you to indicate whether accurate **55.0%**
Allowed you to talk **without interrupting**	Interrupted you **13.4%**	Did not interrupt you directly but cut your responses short by not giving you enough time **22.1%**	Did not interrupt and allowed time to express thoughts fully **64.4%**
Relationship Development			
Communicated **concern** or intention to help	Did not communicate intention to help/concern via words or actions **5.4%**	Words OR actions conveyed intention to help/concern **28.4%**	Actions AND words conveyed intention to help/concern **66.2%**
Non-verbal behavior enriched communication (e.g., eye contact, posture)	Non-verbal behavior was negative or interfered with communication **9.5%**	Non-verbal behavior demonstrated attentiveness **50.7%**	Non-verbal behavior facilitated effective communication **39.9%**
Acknowledged your emotions appropriately	Did not acknowledge your emotions **9.5%**	Attempted to acknowledge emotions **51.7%**	Responded to your emotions in ways that made you feel better **38.8%**
Was **accepting/non-judgmental**	Expressed judgment **1.4%**	Did not express judgment but did not demonstrate respect either **28.1%**	Demonstrated respect towards you **70.5%**
Used words you understood and/or explained **jargon**	Jargon made it difficult to understand **4.0%**	Used jargon occasionally but did not significantly interfere with understanding **23.0%**	Provided no opportunity for misunderstanding by avoiding or explaining jargon **73.0%**

Fig. 2.8 Describing OSCE data for a cohort of trainees. Shown for each OSCE checklist item, the distribution of ratings for a class of third year medical students ($n = 160$)

Table 2.15 Psychometric qualities of OSCE results

	Definition, Key Questions	Enhancement Strategies
Reliability & Internal Consistency	Measures consistency and precision of an assessment tool. If learners underwent the same exam without any interim interventions, would the results be the same? How similar did trainees perform in the different stations? Typically one uses Cronbach's alpha to determine the level of internal consistency (a Cronbach's alpha between .60 and .80 is considered adequate for formative assessments, an alpha of .80 or more is necessary for promotion decisions). Typical sources for unreliability are: □ item differences within cases (case specificity) □ case differences in the use of the rating form □ differences within individual raters in how they applied the rating form □ differences between raters in how they applied the rating form	□ Sufficiently large sample size • of learners • of cases (e.g., samples of communication abilities) □ Clear, easy-to-use rating forms □ Training of raters □ Strong evidence of test item importance □ Elimination of items that are responsible for reducing the OSCEs reliability
Intra-Rater Reliability	Measures consistency of individual raters over time. If a rater would evaluate the same performance a second time, would the result be the same? Contextual differences (e.g., live versus video-taped encounter vs. a video-taped encounter), are expected to influence these estimates of reliability. Nonetheless, if the rating forms are reliable, we would expect to see substantial correlations.	□ Initial selection of raters who are consistent □ Rater training (including feedback on the correlations of assessments of the same video-taped case at different times)
Inter-Rater Reliability	Measures consistency among different raters. If several raters observe the same learner's performance, are their ratings of the performance in agreement?	□ Initial selection of raters who are consistent □ Rater training (including feedback on the level of agreement with other raters of the same real or video-taped encounter)
Validity	Determines whether an OSCE assesses what it is set out to measure (e.g., communication skills, primary care skills). There are multiple types of validity. • Face and content validity (Does it look right?) • Convergent/divergent validity (Does it compare to other measures as it should?) • Discriminant validity (Does it differentiate between training levels or other learner characteristics) • Predictive validity (Does it predict future behavior	□ Re-examination of the blueprint

and peer ratings, etc.)? And ultimately, are checklist scores predictive of actual clinical performance and outcomes?

Standard Setting

Setting standards for pass/fail examinations is both an art and a science. The core issues are determining the appropriate developmental level, and then exploring how to use score cut-offs to divide learners into those that meet those standards and those that do not. For high stakes examinations, many psychometricians and medical education experts recommend absolute or criterion-referenced cut-offs (i.e., scores that reflect the ability to competently perform specific skills and behaviors). Experts review the "test" (OSCE rating form and cases) content and determine a "passing" score. More complicated methods are also available (Boulet et al. 2003 [review]; Kilminster and Roberts 2004; Krumer et al. 2003).

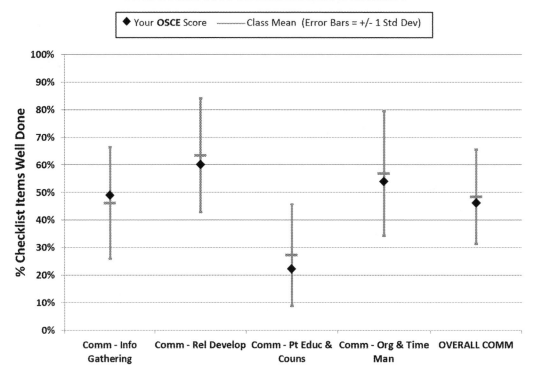

Fig. 2.9 Sample report card illustrating the OSCE performance of an individual learner (following our example General Internal Medicine Residency OSCE). Scores are reported as percentage checklist items "well done" and reflect individual performance across 10 OSCE cases relative to a cohort of 24 OSCE participants (first year residents, in this example)

An alternative is to use relative standards or norm-referenced standards, where a certain percentage of the lowest-performing OSCE participants "fail" (e.g., those with a score in the bottom decile or the bottom 20 %). The obvious problem with this approach is that while the pass/fail cut-off often stays the same, the sample of OSCE participants may vary in their performance over time (a score in the bottom decile in a class of stellar students might be comparable to an average score in a class with greater variation in their skills). This approach also requires that at least some trainees "fail."

Standard setting policy decisions are judgments made by experts. Formal standard setting procedures can assist in ensuring that cut-off scores reflect a consensus among relevant responsible educators. A variety of standard setting processes have been described for performance-based assessments, each with its own underlying assumptions and requirements (Downing et al. 2006). While exams given on a very large scale can afford—both financially and with respect to numbers of subjects and experts—to go through rigorous standard setting procedures, most smaller-scale projects cannot. Therefore most school or program-based summative OSCEs end up using an approach that combines normative, criterion-based, and practical considerations to setting pass/fail cut-offs.

At NYU we use this combined approach for setting cut-offs to identify students who fail our comprehensive clinical skills exam (CCSE), a summative 8-case OSCE required after the core clerkship year. Through rigorous training of raters and refinement of our checklists and patient note rating processes we are able to obtain internally consistent assessments of the four competence areas assessed in the exam (communication skills, history gathering, physical exam, and clinical reasoning as reflected in the patient note). These scores are normally distributed around a mean score between 50 and 60 % and therefore we can identify students at both the upper and lower ends of the spectrum. We have decided that performing well on one competency does not compensate for performing poorly on another. Therefore we report the competency scores separately, taking what is called a non-compensatory approach (Sadler 2005). We then set a normative passing cut-off at the lowest decile for each competency. Students in this lowest decile across two or more competencies are identified, and then all students who "fail" communication skills alone (because we have found that this is predictive of failure on the USMLE Step II CS exam) are added to this list. Students' scores that fall close to the threshold (above and below) are further scrutinized to better make pass/fail decisions. Finally, any student who received a "would not recommend to a friend or family" global rating from more than one SP is added to the list because we have found this identifies additional students who go on to struggle with communication issues clinically and on other OSCEs. Our list of students who fail the exam is based also on our capacity to provide adequate remediation. Remediation strategies are discussed further in Chap. 3 of this book.

Reporting Results

If the OSCE is used solely for training, performance feedback is essential. Even if the OSCE has evaluative purposes, students want and highly value feedback on their performance. Because of the need to keep the content of the OSCE stations secure, there may be limitations on how detailed such reports can be. Training program faculty need to know how learners performed. By identifying those areas of consistent weakness across learners, the curriculum can be modified to enhance learners' clinical performance in the future. Figure 2.9 provides an example of an OSCE score report. Whether in the form of a table or with the help of graphs, learners need to know what scores they achieved and how they compared with their peers. Learners can be encouraged not only to compare their scores with those received by peers but also to explore their relative strengths and weaknesses, noting differences among how they performed within and across particular domains. We aspire to design feedback reports to be easily understood and build in opportunities to develop action plans and ongoing guidance to learners as part of the feedback process.

Longitudinal Educational Database

OSCEs generate a wealth of data and can be combined with data from other sources (faculty ratings, exam scores, self-assessments, even clinical and patient data) over time to track and monitor and understand the development of competence. You can work with your local Institutional Review Board to develop opportunities for obtaining consent from learners to combine those data not just for program evaluation purposes but also for research purposes—to answer both anticipated and unanticipated questions about the longitudinal process of becoming competent professionals. A student or trainee "registry" can be established, just like a patient registry, in which all students or trainees are asked to provide permission for their routinely collected educational data to be linked and compiled in an educational database. Such data, once linked and stored, should be de-identified, that is, all identifiers should be stripped from the data except for the unique ID generated for the purpose of the database. Creation of this database can provide invaluable data on performance across domains over time and also help establish the quality of assessments made throughout the curriculum.

Best Practices: Managing and Analyzing OSCE Data

- Plan for and monitor the quality of data entry and management; use unique identifiers to maintain confidentiality and make sure data are backed up and maintained securely.
- Explore the quality of the data in terms of reliability estimates of internal consistency (Cronbach's alpha) before calculating summary scores.
- Calculate OSCE scores based on performance within domains across stations, considering the structure of the data (response options) and how best to derive summaries (percentage well done, average of scaled items, nonparametric methods if necessary).
- Report performance data to learners in ways that are understandable and constructive.
- Consider how to mine the wealth of educational data available by creating registries and organizing and linking data and information from many relevant sources.

Step 10

Develop a Case Library and Institutionalize OSCEs

The first OSCE requires an especially great deal of effort. However, as a set of cases is created, materials developed, a cadre of SPs recruited, and the team involved gets more experience, organizing OSCEs becomes much easier. By developing a case library such the one exemplified in Fig. 2.10, one can greatly reduce preparations for subsequent OSCEs. It is useful to maintain a library in electronic (backed-up!) and paper format and to make sure that the latest versions of the cases (and training notes) are archived. It is also helpful to maintain a database of SPs and their contact information, and of any evaluative data that may have accumulated for each station. In this way, one can determine whether cases need to be tweaked and whether SPs should be invited back.

Given that licensure exams now include performance-based assessments, and that the ACGME and other accrediting agencies now strongly advocate for the use of OSCEs, it makes sense for organizers to invest energy in institutionalizing OSCEs. Below are some tips for making OSCEs part of the institutional culture.

	Case		SP Characteristics		Nature of Encounter			Skills Assessed					
ID	Name	Details	Age	Gender	Acute v Chronic	Presenting Condition	Nature of Visit	Comm	Hx Gather	Phys Exam	Tx Plan & Man	Other	Last Used
1	Work Rounds	Sub-intern and team conduct work rounds	58	F	Acute	Metastatic Breast Ca	Rounds	✓			✓	Precepting	2009
2	Depression	Precept MS IV on ambulatory rotation	64	M	Chronic	Depression	Ongoing	✓	✓		✓	Precepting	2011
3	New Diagnosis	Pt hospitalized while on vacation	55	M	Acute	High BP, Afib	New Visit	✓	✓	✓	✓	System-based practice	2009
54	Diarrhea	Pt calls complaining of diarrhea	35	M	Chronic	Diarrhea	Ongoing	✓	✓		✓	Phone Skills	2010
55	Shoulder Pain	Pt diagnosed with RCC 8 mos ago	62	F	Acute	Metastatic Renal Cell Ca	New Onset	✓	✓	✓	✓		2009
56	Stomach Ache	Pt complaining of stomach pain; worse with GAD	32	F	Chronic	GAD	Ongoing	✓	✓	✓	✓		2011
57	Cholesterol	Pt with hx of HTN and hyperlipemia; noncompliant	45	M	Chronic	HTN, Hyperlipidemia	New Visit	✓	✓		✓		2007
58	Chest Pain	Pt with hx of NIDDM and HTN presents with chest pain	56	F	Acute	NIDDM, HTN	New Visit	✓	✓	✓	✓	Inter-profnl Collab	2010

Fig. 2.10 Snapshot of OSCE cases and characteristics stored in 120-case bank. A database aids in organizing and tracking use of cases and in developing an OSCE blueprint such as that shown in Fig. 2.4

Best Practices: Building Institutional Capacity

- Save all material on an institutional server.
- Create a collaborative interdisciplinary OSCE committee that meets regularly.
- Invite institutional opinion leaders and early adaptors from various departments to observe, help out, stop by.
- Disseminate reports widely.
- Talk about the OSCEs all year round (and with humor!).
- Get the OSCE into your departmental budget.
- Apply for research and program enhancement grants.
- Publish and present experience/findings locally, nationally, and internationally.

Remediation of Learners Who Perform Poorly on an OSCE

Adina Kalet, Linda Tewksbury, Jennifer Ogilvie, Lynn Buckvar-Keltz, Barbara Porter, and Sandra Yingling

Data from well-designed OSCEs help educators identify trainees with gaps in their core clinical skills. Yet there is little consensus on effective remediation strategies for individuals who perform poorly. Experts stress that it is important to clearly delineate the implications and consequences of learner failure in any performance assessment (Cleland et al. 2005; Sayer et al. 2002; Segal et al. 1999; Schwartz et al. 1998) and assert that successful remediation requires approaches tailored to identified deficits (Hauer et al. 2009). By definition, learner remediation must have a reasonable chance of leading to an improvement in clinical competence. Table 3.1 breaks the remediation process down into manageable steps. Effective remediation first of all requires good data (see Chap. 2, Step 9 for an in-depth discussion of standard setting). Also crucial, to engage meaningfully in and gain life-long benefit from remediation, learners must have or develop the capacity to accurately self-assess and self-regulate learning.

A. Kalet, M.D., M.P.H. (✉)
Department of Medicine, Division of General Internal Medicine, Section of Primary Care, New York University School of Medicine, New York, NY, USA
e-mail: Adina.Kalet@nyumc.org

L. Tewksbury, M.D.
Department of Pediatrics, New York University School of Medicine, New York, NY, USA

J. Ogilvie, M.D., F.A.C.S.
Department of Surgery, New York University School of Medicine, New York, NY, USA

L. Buckvar-Keltz, M.D.
Office of Student Affairs, New York University School of Medicine, New York, NY, USA

B. Porter, M.D., M.P.H.
Department of Medicine, Bellevue Hospital Center, New York, NY, USA

S. Yingling, Ph.D.
Office of Medical Education, New York University School of Medicine, New York, NY, USA

Initiating the Remediation Process

Not surprisingly, trainees are usually very upset upon hearing they have failed an OSCE. A structured first meeting between the student and faculty member responsible for remediation, which allows enough time for discussion of feelings, a student's self-assessment, and a careful review of data from the exam, is reassuring to the student and will most likely to lead to an effective remediation. Depending on the nature of the OSCE (low stakes/formative versus high stakes/summative), the remediation process can be more or less comprehensive. For a low-stakes exam, a brief individual feedback session, with videotape review if available, may be sufficient. Table 3.2 provides outline for a comprehensive intake meeting in a high-stakes situation. We schedule 1.5 h for this initial session.

Using detailed data from the OSCE in remediation is invaluable because it helps "break down" learner resistance to the process, builds accurate self-assessment skills, and if necessary provides the support for documentation for disciplinary actions. These data may include the various sources of information listed in Table 3.3.

Characterizing the Difficulty

There are a host of reasons learners fail an OSCE. The most common reasons for failure are summarized in Table 3.4[1] in order of frequency.

Once the faculty facilitator and the learner come to a negotiated agreement on one or more areas of difficulty, a contract or individualized remediation plan (IRP) should be drafted and follow-up plans made. This document (see Fig. 3.1 for an example) should evolve as the remediation process proceeds

---

[1] Kalet A. et.al. (manuscript in progress). Our experience with clinical skills remediation for three consecutive classes of medical students, 2007–2009. During this time period, 53 of 500 students failed. Sample learning diagnoses are listed from most remediable to least.

Table 3.1 Steps in the remediation process

1. *Gather and carefully review objective data of performance*
2. *Obtain student self-assessment and provide feedback based on objective data*
3. *Assess for nonacademic issues*
4. *Make an educational diagnosis*
5. *Formulate an individualized learning plan with diagnosis specific remediation strategies* (think creatively about available resources!)
6. *Make a plan to follow-up on progress and measure*

Table 3.2 OSCE remediation initial diagnostic interview

☐ *Statement of expectations*
☐ *Learner self-assessment*
☐ *Assessment of exam-specific performance issues*
☐ *Educational history* Including screening for verbal and nonverbal learning disabilities, attention deficit disorders, language fluency
☐ *Assessment of professionalism* e.g., learner attitudes toward the OSCE, accountability for performance
☐ *Screening for situational stressors*
☐ *Screening for common psychiatric illness* e.g., depression, anxiety, bipolar disorder, eating disorders, substance abuse

Table 3.3 Learner data useful for remediation

☐ *Performance across OSCE cases compared to the group means*
☐ *Performance by case*
☐ *Post SP encounter notes*
☐ *SP comments* (after prescreening)
☐ *Videotape of the encounter*
☐ *Other evaluation data available* e.g., academic record, clerkship comments

Table 3.4 Areas of difficulty leading to poor OSCE performance

1. *Preexisting academic issues*
   - Learning disabilities
   - Poor academic track-record especially on stressful clinical rotations
   - Nontraditional educational paths such as learners with discontinuous training (e.g., MD-PhD programs) or transfer from other programs (e.g., accelerated BS-MD programs)
2. *Isolated clinical skills deficit* i.e., specific area(s) of weakness such as knowledge base, communication, reasoning, or problem-solving skills
3. *Metacognitive or specific testing issues*
   - Time management or organizational difficulties
   - Insufficient preparation or poor understanding of the exam
   - Performance anxiety
4. *Extenuating psychological factors*
   - Anxiety
   - Depression
   - Situation-specific duress
5. *Nonverbal learning disorders* e.g., long-standing social awkwardness, autism spectrum disorders
6. *Professionalism issues* i.e., learner does not know or agree with health professional tenets and values; paranoid, combative, or defiant personality style or frank personality disorder

and new light is shed on the student's strengths and weaknesses. Keeping the IRP updated provides an efficient communication tool among the members of the remediation team and keeps the student actively engaged in the process.

In Table 3.5 we list remediation strategies we use regularly. Relevant references include Pinsky and Wipf (2000) for videotape review, Bowen (2006) and Croskerry (2003) for clinical reasoning and critical thinking, and Kogan et al. (2009) for direct observation with feedback. The primary purpose of any strategy is to enhance the learner's awareness of deficits and enabling them to improve their clinical performance. Strategies used will depend on the issues, available resources, and the learner's willingness to explore difficult issues.

Who Should Participate in Learner Remediation?

The most effective facilitators of clinical competence remediation are likely to be, but not restricted to, experienced clinician educators. Table 3.6 lists examples of the experts and specialists who we have found are invaluable to the effort.

Faculty Development for Remediation

The institutional capacity to remediate learners who fail a high-stakes OSCE is entirely dependent on the number, commitment, and expertise of the faculty members available to participate. Faculty members who enjoy working with learners one-on-one, are good listeners; skillful at giving effective feedback, knowledgeable about learning disorders and psychiatric diagnoses and who are interested in the development of clinical competence are ideally suited for this work but may need additional training to maximize their effectiveness. Table 3.7 lists learning objectives for faculty development in clinical skills remediation. Educators specifically interested in reading more about defining behavioral measures of clinical competence are referred to Quirk (2006).

Make-Up OSCE

A remediation program, to be effective, must culminate in a measure of learner performance. In remediation for high-stakes exams, we require students to participate in and pass a four-station OSCE, which is a mix of cases repeated from the

Fig. 3.1 Example individualized remediation plan

	Learning Goals	Strategies	Evidence of Improvement
1.	Improve my rapport-building skills, especially non-verbal expressions of attention and concern.	Practice with an SP until I can do this consistently (2-3 sessions).	Perform adequately on Remediation OSCE.
2.	Improve my clinical reasoning so that I can include more pertinent negative historical and physical exam facts in a patient note.	Write up 10 practice cases and review these with Dr. X. Respond to feedback by demonstrating commitment to learning.	Perform above the threshold on Remediation OSCE.
3.	Explore my attitudes about patients who are seeking pain medication.	Write and discuss 3 brief essays: Physicians' attitudes toward pain management in terminally ill patients; Barriers to adequate pain relief in chronic pain syndromes; Ethical issues when treating pain.	By the Remediation OSCE, Dr. X will be satisfied that I have explored my own attitudes and beliefs in this area.

Table 3.5 Selected remediation strategies

1. *Self-directed videotape review (VTR)* Using a blank OSCE checklist the learner rates his/her performance on one or two videotaped encounters from the actual OSCE, summarizes his/her findings from the VTR, and reviews these documents with a faculty adviser

2. *Faculty-facilitated videotape review* In learners who demonstrate poor self-awareness of their difficulties a structured, faculty-facilitated VTR can help the student recognize areas of difficulty

3. *SP practice with feedback* A learner with very specific communication difficulties can benefit from scheduled sessions with an SP experienced in giving feedback, to practice the skills

4. *Clinical reasoning practice* Learners are assigned reading about the clinical reasoning/critical thinking process to enhance metacognitive awareness and then practice with paper or Web-based cases

5. *Direct observation with real patients*

6. *Physical exam workshops* Can be done in groups with a faculty or resident facilitator; active practice and discussion about findings is critical to success

7. *Reflective writing* Brief assignments asking learner to reflect on attitudes and beliefs expressed or demonstrated which do not align with medical professionalism or effective patient care

8. *Directed readings* Relevant when there is an isolated knowledge deficit or lack of understanding of specific principles such as the tenets of medical professionalism or standards of treatment (e.g., substance abuse)

9. *Work with a specialist* e.g., referrals for psychiatric assessment, interpersonal skills coaching, performance anxiety strategies, learning/organization support, and career advice

Table 3.6 Experts and specialists who can contribute to learner remediation

1. *Clinical educators* Best suited to conduct the initial assessment, work with learners on clinical reasoning or physical examination deficits, monitor remediation process, and make a final outcome determination

2. *Communication skills coach* Learners with isolated communication deficits or professionalism issues benefit from working with a coach familiar with the health care environment and skilled with behaviorally focused coaching approaches

3. *Drama therapist/SP trainer/experienced SP* Learners with communication skills deficits or performance anxiety benefit from practice with feedback and coaching

4. *Learning specialist/studying or executive function coach* Learners with a long-standing history of uneven academic performance, atypical organizational strategies, unusual study strategies, or who don't "read for pleasure" may have undiagnosed learning disabilities

5. *Psychiatrist/psychologist* (when a psychiatric diagnosis is suspected or already established)

6. *Role model* A respected member of the clinical field related to the learner's interests can be effective at encouraging the student to engage in the remediation enthusiastically

Table 3.7 Learning objectives for clinical skills remediation faculty development

Clinical educators conducting remediation with learners who fail an OSCE should be able to…
1. Interpret quantitative and qualitative data regarding the competence of individual medical trainees
2. Define clinical competence in a behaviorally specific, measurable manner
3. List common areas of difficulty for trainees struggling to pass an OSCE
4. Discuss the role of normal adult development in assessing clinical competence development
5. Describe the screening process needed to identify a learning disability or attention deficit disorder
6. Demonstrate the ability to screen for common psychiatric issues that may manifest as or coexist with clinical incompetence
7. Make defendable judgments regarding clinical competence
8. Conduct an effective, satisfying, and growth promoting remediation process
9. Document a remediation process that is meaningful and addresses legal and regulatory requirements
10. Explore personal attitudes and beliefs which inhibit effective identification and remediation of learners who struggle to achieve minimal competence
11. Understand that on rare occasions a student may fail the make-up exam

OSCE they failed and new cases. Because reliability of a four-station OSCE is predictably poorer than one with more cases we determine the outcome of this exam using standards established in the larger exam and take into account findings from a detailed review of the student's performance. Each case is videotaped or directly observed by a faculty familiar with the student.

Considerations When Documenting Remediation

Detailed documentation of the remediation process is important both to ensure communication among the remediation team and to provide evidence to support promotion decisions. At the minimum, programs should keep track of learner's data on OSCEs, standards for pass/fail decisions, IRPs, and document date and time of meetings between learners and members of the remediation team. We have found it helpful to write a brief narrative summary of each session with a learner, documenting updates to the IRP, and agreed upon next steps. Depending on the local law and regulatory environment, schools and training programs have obligations and responsibilities to keep written records of the evidence that learners have demonstrated training stage appropriate competence. Remediation team leaders should familiarize themselves with the government, accreditation agency (ACGME, LCME), and institutional documentation requirements that may apply to the remediation process. In the United States, in addition to documentation requirements for the purposes of accreditation, there is relevant federal law that seeks to protect the privacy of students, patients, and employees by limiting access to records (the Family Educational Rights and Privacy Act of 1974 [FERPA]; see www2.ed.gov/policy/gen/guid/fpco/ferpa/index.html) and personal health information (the Health Insurance Portability and Accountability Act of 1996 [HIPAA]; see www.hhs.gov/ocr/privacy/hipaa/understanding/index.html). Balancing the needs to document a complex process in a meaningful way and understanding the legal environment will help each program design an efficient record keeping process which serves both the program and the learners. On rare occasions, a student may not be successful in their remediation. The institution must be able to accept this outcome while supporting the student with psychologic support and career advice.

Remediation of learners who perform poorly on an OSCE provides a unique opportunity to explore the underlying reason(s) for substandard clinical skills and to intervene in a highly impactful manner. Although many of these learners are challenging, there is rich opportunity for professional and personal growth in the student as well as development of a therapeutic alliance between the learner and remediation specialist(s). In our experience, most students gain valuable insight regarding their difficulties, are committed to working with the remediation team, and successfully complete the make-up academic exercises. Work remains to be done regarding the identification of the most effective, efficient, and least costly remediation techniques for the various subtypes of problems leading to failure on clinical skills examinations.

Sondra Zabar, Angela Burgess, Kathleen Hanley,
and Elizabeth Krajic Kachur

Beyond the OSCE: Evaluation Clinical Skills Using Unannounced Standardized Patients

Although the use of standardized patients (SPs) is widely used in assessment, the vast majority of SP exercises/exams involve announced encounters in which the learners know that they are interacting with a simulated patient. Objective structured clinical examinations (OSCEs) are considered a gold standard for assessing clinical skills, but their overtly contrived nature may limit their ability to capture the true behavior of medical professionals (Ozuah and Reznik 2007). The use of unannounced standardized patients (USPs) is a relatively new but increasingly used method for evaluating the competence of medical professionals (Glassman et al. 2000; Rethans et al. 2007). USP encounters do not have the artificial time constraints of OSCEs, and USPs can evaluate subjects in a real clinic setting.

USPs have been used to assess trainees as well as practitioners across the health professions, including nursing (Carney and Ward 1998), optometry (Shah et al. 2007), and a range of medical specialties, from primary care (Culver

S. Zabar, M.D. (✉)
Department of Medicine, Division of General Internal Medicine,
Section of Primary Care, New York University School of Medicine,
550 First Avenue, BCD D401, New York, NY 10016, USA
e-mail: sondra.zabar@nyumc.org

A. Burgess
Program for Medical Education Innovations and Research,
New York University School of Medicine,
New York, NY, USA

K. Hanley, M.D.
Department of Medicine, Division of General Internal Medicine,
Section of Primary Care, New York University School of Medicine,
New York, NY, USA

E.K. Kachur, Ph.D.
Medical Education Development, National and International
Consulting, New York, NY, USA

et al. 2009) to emergency medicine (Zabar et al. 2009). The published literature describes using USPs to assess clinical skills (e.g., [in residents], Ozuah and Reznik 2008a, b) or the efficacy of educational interventions. The performance of clinicians visited by USPs may be compared with that of a group who did not receive an intervention (control group) or to their own performance in announced standardized patient encounters. Intervention studies (e.g., Casebeer et al. 1999) determine the success of an educational initiative, generally by comparing performance with USPs before and after the intervention. Other studies explore the feasibility and validity of USPs compared to chart reviews and clinical vignettes (Peabody et al. 2000).

USPs can also be used to evaluate the clinical microsystem. A clinic's commitment to becoming a patient-centered medical home is as important to health outcomes as the skills of its physicians. USPs can rate the performance of medical assistants, the ease of navigating the clinic, and the functioning of the clinic care team (Peabody et al. 2004; Zabar et al. 2009). USPs easily documents adherence to national patient safety standards, such as hand washing and patient identification. USPs can also observe a clinic's level of patient centeredness (Epstein et al. 2005). Because they undergo every level of the patient experience, USPs are versatile judges of health centers.

Health professional schools that conduct OSCEs are poised to incorporate a USP program into their curriculum, as much of the infrastructure required to perform the two assessments is similar, such as SP/rater training and case development. Since USPs are integrated into an already established clinic setting, costs are limited to compensation for the actors. Hourly rates for standardized patients range from $15 to $25 per hour, and most USP visits last 2–4 h. Additional USP requirements include close collaboration with administrators in the clinical setting.

USP programs are not without potential difficulties. There is a risk that USPs will be detected, which can undermine the effectiveness of the program. If a medical professional realizes (s)he is interacting with a USP, he or she may not behave in natural manner. Consequently, the data collected still may not reflect a clinician's true skills. Matching USPs with the intended clinician can be complicated in some health centers, particularly those that do not assign patients to specific providers. Constant communication with scheduling coordinators is necessary to ensure that USPs interact with the correct clinicians. There is also the concern that USP visits hinder productivity by taking up trainee patient time. However the few number of visits needed to evaluate the clinical system and provider performance is usually seen as worth the investment by hospital and educational leadership.

USP Staffing Needs

USP projects can be a major undertaking, and as with most other educational projects, collaboration within and across specialties, even across disciplines can only enrich the process. While it is necessary to have strong leaders who believe in the benefits of such comprehensive assessment programs, many other individuals are needed for adequate planning, preparation, and implementation. Table 4.1 details the additional roles that USP projects typically require beyond those detailed in for OSCE administration Table 2.1.

Implementing a USP Project

Specific tasks involved in planning to integrate USP visits in a clinical setting are detailed in Table 4.2, a modification of the worksheet for assigning OSCE responsibilities and creating timelines (Fig. 2.3, Appendix C).

Cases

USP and OSCE case development follow the same basic principles (see Chap. 2, Step 4, "Develop Cases and Stations"). Many OSCE cases can easily be adopted to be

Table 4.1 USP staffing needs (see also: Table 2.1)

Roles	Key characteristics	# Needed
Leader	▪ Strong motivation to develop and implement project ▪ Well connected to procure resources ▪ Can establish collaborative relationship with hospital/clinic leadership ▪ Able to communicate well and create a team spirit	One or more
Planner	▪ Understands logistics of implementing USP (case development, project location) ▪ Can entertain multiple options for solving problems	One or more
Coordinator	▪ Can implement USP-related tasks (e.g., scheduling, SP recruitment, data entry) ▪ Able to communicate well ▪ Good at troubleshooting and problem solving	One or more (depending on scope)
Clinical Administrator	▪ Can obtain fake medical records ▪ Able to assess workflow to incorporate USP with no detection	Usually one
Trainer	▪ Understands USP roles and case requirements ▪ Has teaching skills (e.g., provides constructive feedback) and can manage psychosocial impact of case portrayals ▪ Able to communicate well and create a team spirit ▪ Is sensitive to the special stresses inherent in USP work	One or more (depending on scope)
SPs	▪ Committed to standardization of their case portrayal (i.e., not expressing their personal creativity) ▪ Comfortable enacting their particular medical case (i.e., not getting too involved emotionally) ▪ Interested in taking on "educational" responsibilities ▪ Able to tolerate the open-ended nature of USP visits (can last from 30 min to 3 h or more) ▪ Comfortable to be among individuals who have true medical conditions and may be in emotional or physical distress (e.g., heart attack in an emergency room) ▪ Able to change appearance if using one clinical site ▪ Clear about USP goals and performance standards ▪ Committed to fair performance assessments (e.g., understands personal rater style and biases) ▪ Effective provider of post-encounter feedback	At least one per case, consider cross-trained alternates
Data Manager	▪ Can enter performance data ▪ Understands USP process ▪ Committed to accuracy	At least one
Data Analyst	▪ Understands USP process ▪ Has psychometric skills ▪ Understands end-users of results (e.g., learners, program)	At least one
Program Evaluator	▪ Understands USP process ▪ Is familiar with evaluation models (e.g., pre-/posttesting) ▪ Can develop and analyze program evaluations (e.g., surveys, focus groups)	At least one

Table 4.2 Breakdown of USP responsibilities

	Initial planning
3–4 months before planned start of USP project	■ Obtain permission from and initiate partnership with clinic administrators ■ Decide on format (e.g., number of cases, time frame) ■ Create a blueprint (identify competencies to be assessed) ■ Develop cases ■ Identify single or multiple locations of project ■ Recruit staff (for administrative tasks, scheduling) ■ Identify each step of USP visit (check in procedure, insurance, medical record) ■ Decide on USP recruitment and training schedule ■ Communicate with learners (explain nature of project, get consent for USP visits) ■ Clarify budget (e.g., USP costs, recording equipment)
	Material, USP, and visit preparations
3 months to 1 week before first USP visit	■ Develop USP materials (e.g., USP instructions, rating forms) ■ Recruit USPs ■ Create medical records and unique case demographics ■ Prepare props (e.g., fake pill bottles, inhalers, charts, insurance cards) ■ Train USPs ■ Organize practice visits ("dress rehearsals") ■ Consider videotaping USP training sessions ■ Consider audio-recording USP visits ■ Create schedule for practice/clinic visits ■ Send demographic info (name, address, DoB) to clinic director and to USP
	USP Administration
Day of USP visit	■ Provide USP with audio recorder and transportation funds, if necessary ■ Direct USP to practice/clinic site ■ Provide rating form post-visit ■ Debrief USP post-visit with the help of the rating form ■ Consider audio- or videotaping debriefing session ■ Plan periodic group debriefing sessions with USPs to share experiences and control for desirable and undesirable case adjustments
	Post-USP tasks
Days to weeks after USP visit	■ Organize rating forms and clinic materials by case ■ Arrange for USP payment ■ Enter data and evaluation results ■ Survey learners for detection ■ Report evaluation data (e.g., report cards) ■ Organize materials for future reference (e.g., forms, videos) ■ Report on experience internally and externally (e.g., presentations, articles)

used in USP visits. To prevent detection, it is crucial to make sure that USP cases are representative of the patient population served by the providers one plans to evaluate. A sample USP case and corresponding checklist, designed for an urban community clinic, are included at the end of this book as Appendices N and O.

Recruitment

The number of USPs required depends on the number of cases in the program, the number of clinicians involved, and the duration of the program. Medical schools are the best places to recruit USPs, since they work with actors who already have experience as standardized patients. The most qualified standardized patients will possess acting talent, punctuality, communication skills, and the ability to adapt to unpredictable situations.

Training

USP training sessions are similar to OSCE training exercises. Trainings can be divided into three sessions. During the first session, the USP program coordinator explains the purpose and logistics of the program to USPs. USPs should then read the case instructions aloud with the USP coordinator. After it is clear that the USPs fully understand their role, they practice the case, taking on the patient role while the coordinator assumes the role of physician. The second training focuses on teaching USPs to complete the evaluation forms. The coordinator shows a presentation about the correct way to observe, categorize, and document clinicians' behavior. To practice completing the evaluation, the USPs should watch OSCE encounters and evaluate learners' skills. During the final training session, the USPs can role-play the case with an attending physician or chief resident to learn the pacing of a medical interview. The USP coordinator can discreetly bring the USPs to the clinic before their first visits to prepare USPs for navigating the area.

Clinic Location and Visits

Before any visits are planned, program leaders must get permission from clinic administrators to conduct the program. They should speak to members of the finance office to learn how to prevent USP visits from being billed as real visits and appearing in clinic audits.

The USP coordinator should visit the clinic during a busy day to observe its layout. He or she should note the location of the registration desk, exam rooms, and other relevant areas (finance desk, pharmacy, etc.) The coordinator must observe where patients must go to check in, pay, encounter doctors, and get prescriptions and referrals. The coordinator will be better prepared to train USPs to navigate the clinic if he or she is aware of the path real patients travel.

The program team then identifies the unique characteristics of the clinic that will receive USPs. In some clinics, it is possible to schedule appointments with a specific doctor; in others, patients are assigned doctors in a first come, first serve basis. The USP coordinator needs to work with the clinic's patient coordinator to develop a system that will ensure USPs are sent to the correct physicians. The patient coordinator should also be responsible for entering USPs' demographic information into the clinic's computer system. The USP coordinator can develop a process and deadline for sending the demographic information for each visit.

The USP coordinator collaborates with the patient coordinator to develop the USP visit schedule. The USP coordinator chooses dates and times for USP visits and sends them to the patient coordinator for approval. The patient coordinator approves the requests if the appointments are available and can suggest edits to the USP coordinator's selections if there are scheduling conflicts.

After the schedule is finalized, the USP coordinator asks USPs to sign up for visits. On the day of a visit, the USP coordinator should meet with the USP before the visit begins to give him or her an audio recorder. USP visits should be recorded in order to validate the checklist data. After the USP gets the recorder, he or she enters the clinic.

The USP should invent an excuse to avoid getting labs ordered by a physician. For example, he or she can say they have to go back to work or just ate. The USP should hold onto any paperwork he or she is given (prescriptions, referrals, etc.) and return it to the USP coordinator after the visit.

Post-visit

After the visit is complete, the USP meets with the coordinator to complete the evaluation. The coordinator reviews the evaluation for missing data and inconsistencies, then performs a debriefing session, where qualitative data about the visit is discussed. Topics raised during the debriefing include the atmosphere of the clinic, the conduct of the resident and/ or medical assistants, and the degree of difficulty in navigating the clinic. Debriefing sessions should also explore facilitators and barriers to patient care. When the visit is complete, the USP signs an invoice.

Budgeting

The USP coordinator can keep track of the program costs in an Excel spreadsheet. All training and visit costs for each USP should be documented and updated frequently to ensure the program stays within the budget. The spreadsheet should include the name and contact information of each USP, list every date each USP worked, and include the amount USPs were paid for each visit or training session. Excel can calculate the total program costs and the average costs per visit. For example, the NYU School of Medicine USP program costs about $120 per visit.

Learner, Microsystem, and Programmatic Evaluation

USP visits provide a wealth of information. The program leaders can disseminate a summary report for clinicians on their overall performance across all USP cases. The clinic administrators should receive a summary report of the health care team's performance for patient safety, patient centeredness, screening assessments, and team skills.

USP scores can also be compared to OSCE performance to see how an individual performs in a testing situation versus the "real world" of the clinical environment. The sample evaluation in Fig. 4.1 shows individual and mean cohort primary care resident communication skills as measured in a ten-station OSCE and across multiple USP visits (% checklist items "well done"). As can be seen in the sample report, this particular resident ("Dr. K") actually shows a trend of performing better in USP visits as compared with OSCE encounters.

In our program, USPs were asked to evaluate clinical microsystem as well as clinician performance in 50 visits to primary care providers at an urban community clinic. During each visit, USPs recorded whether the medical assistant greeted the patient within a reasonable time frame; introduced his or herself; wore a visible name tag; washed hands before touching me; measured my height; took my blood pressure; weighed me; and screened for depression. USPs also assessed their general experience with clinic: how easy it was to navigate the system; team functioning; and overall staff professionalism.

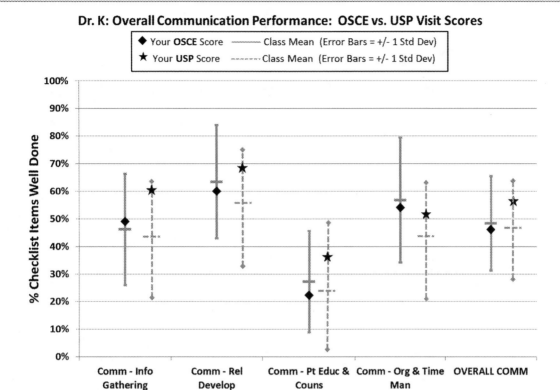

Fig. 4.1 Sample learner feedback report: OSCE versus USP communication performance. Communication sub-competency scores reported: information gathering, relationship development, patient education and counseling, and organization and time management

Clinic administrators then conducted an educational intervention with the medical assistants to improve performance. In preliminary subsequent USP visits post-intervention marked improvements were noted. Clinical microsystems data such as these serve to inform medical directors of critical gaps in patient safety measures, patient satisfaction, and patient centeredness. With specific data on the patient experience, administrators can implement appropriate improvement measures.

Appendix A
Worksheet: OSCE Planning

OSCE Project Name	
OSCE Goals	
Number and Type of Trainees	
Number and Type of Stations	
Potential Timing	
Potential Space	
Budget Available and Potential Funding Sources	
Motivational Strategies	

S. Zabar et al. (eds.), *Objective Structured Clinical Examinations*,
DOI 10.1007/978-1-4614-3749-9, © Springer Science+Business Media New York 2013

Budget items to consider	$ Needed	In Kind	Cost per learner
Space 1 room per station, SP/faculty, and learner meeting areas			
SPs—training and OSCE performance Check for local rates, costs vary depending on location, and simulation task. Ask SPs to arrive ½ h prior to the start of the OSCE and factor early arrival into payment			
Raters—training and rater tasks That is, when faculty raters are used instead of or in addition to SP; consider credit for "teaching" if direct reimbursement of faculty is not possible			
Refreshments Need not be fancy, but can help create a more relaxed atmosphere			
Medical supply Need not be sterile but should be authentic			
Office supply Photocopying forms, pens			
Video equipment and supply Sample learner performance for quality control and future learning activities. Cameras may be purchased (a recommended one-time investment!), rented, or borrowed			
Data entry and report card assembly May be performed by in-house or temporary staff			
Data analysis Faculty/staff with statistical capabilities are vital to an OSCE organization team			
TOTAL			

S. Zabar et al. (eds.), *Objective Structured Clinical Examinations*,
DOI 10.1007/978-1-4614-3749-9, © Springer Science+Business Media New York 2013

OSCE Project Name:	Date:

	Tasks	Individuals Involved	Deadline
	Overall Initial Planning		
3-4 months before the OSCE	• Decide on format (e.g., number of stations, time frame)		
	• Create a blueprint (identify competencies to be assessed)		
	• Decide on what to maintain from previous OSCEs/develop new cases		
	• Identify appropriate OSCE location (stations and assembly rooms)		
	• Recruit staff (for administrative tasks, monitoring, time keeping)		
	• Decide on SP/rater recruitment and training schedule		
	• Communicate with learners (e.g., provide dates/times, explain procedure)		
	• Clarify budget (e.g., SP costs, refreshments)		
	• Consider videotaping		
	Station/Material Preparations		
1 week - 3 months before the OSCE	• Review old station/OSCE materials (e.g., learner/SP instructions, rating forms)		
	• Develop new station/OSCE materials (i.e., content generation and formatting)		
	• Determine SP payment process		
	• Make room arrangements		
	• Recruit SPs		
	• Train SPs		
	• Recruit faculty		
	• Prepare faculty (e.g., circulate station/format information, rater training)		
	• Prepare props (e.g., fake pill bottles and charts)		

General Preparations

1-2 weeks before the OSCE	▪ Order supplies (e.g., paper, folders)		
	▪ Order refreshments		
	▪ Photocopy station materials		
	▪ Assign SPs, faculty and learners (create assignment sheets)		
	▪ Prepare name tags/labels for learners (assign learner IDs)		
	▪ Develop rotation schedules		
	▪ Prepare invoices and necessary paperwork for SP payment		
	▪ Prepare signs (e.g., station numbers, arrows to signal flow)		
	▪ Orient hall monitors and time keepers		

OSCE Administration

day of the OSCE	▪ Prepare stations and assembly rooms (signs, station materials, refreshments)		
	▪ Assign substitutes (if necessary)		
	▪ Orient faculty, SPs and other personnel		
	▪ Position faculty, SPs, hall monitors and time keepers		
	▪ Orient learners (e.g., assign starting station, disseminate name/number labels)		
	▪ Guide learners to individual starting stations		
	▪ Time stations (start, feedback, station changes)		
	▪ Manage emergencies (e.g., equipment breakdown)		
	▪ Assure smooth changeovers of SPs, faculty and learners		
	▪ Reassemble learner group (e.g., for debriefing, program evaluations)		
	▪ Collect and count all forms		
	▪ Clean up stations and assembly rooms		

Post-OSCE Tasks

days to months after the OSCE	▪ Sort out forms		
	▪ Ensure timely SP payment		
	▪ Enter data and evaluation results		
	▪ Analyze data		
	▪ Report evaluation data (e.g., report cards)		
	▪ Report on experience internally and externally (e.g.,		

Appendix D
Worksheet: OSCE Blueprint

	Station		Skills Assessed				Comments
	Case	Content Areas	Comm	History Gathering	Physical Exam	Treatment Mgmt & Plan	
1							
2							
3							
4							
5							
6							
7							
8							
9							
10							

S. Zabar et al. (eds.), *Objective Structured Clinical Examinations*,
DOI 10.1007/978-1-4614-3749-9, © Springer Science+Business Media New York 2013

Appendix E
Worksheet: OSCE Participant Rotation Schedule

This worksheet includes rotation timeslots (columns) for 12 participants in a 12-station OSCE or a 10-station OSCE including two rest stations. To complete the schedule, first fill in the names of the participants in the left-hand column. Add the station numbers across the top blank row (i.e., 1–12 or 1–5, rest, 6–10, rest). Do the same with the next row, except shift the order of the stations by one (i.e., begin with station #2 and end with #1), and continue completing the table in this manner until all the rows are filled. Refer to Fig. 2.6 for a sample completed schedule.

		Rotation (fill in start times)											
Station #		1	2	3	4	5	6	7	8	9	10	11	12
Participant name/ID													

S. Zabar et al. (eds.), *Objective Structured Clinical Examinations*,
DOI 10.1007/978-1-4614-3749-9, © Springer Science+Business Media New York 2013

Appendix F
Sample OSCE Case

A station overview and participant (General Internal Medicine resident, in this case) and SP instructions for the "Medical Error Disclosure" case are included below.

Station overview: MEDICAL ERROR DISCLOSURE

DEVELOPMENT DATE	April 1, 2012
STATION DEVELOPERS	S. Zabar, E. Kachur, K. Hanley, A. Kalet
LEARNERS (intended and potential)	General Internal Medicine residents Also suitable for: Categorical Internal Medicine residents, medical students
OBJECTIVES	To test learners' ability to: 1. Admit an error has been made 2. Express empathy 3. Address patient concerns surrounding an error 4. Reestablish rapport
LOGISTICS	Personnel: Standardized patient, male, early 40s, dressed in street clothing (casual), sitting in chair Room requirements/resources: • 2 Chairs • Medical equipment—none • Other props—none

S. Zabar et al. (eds.), *Objective Structured Clinical Examinations*,
DOI 10.1007/978-1-4614-3749-9, © Springer Science+Business Media New York 2013

Resident instructions: MEDICAL ERROR DISCLOSURE

PATIENT INFORMATION

Name: John McCoy
Age: 42
Marital status: single, never married
Occupation: musician/waiter

REASON FOR ENCOUNTER

Patient initiated visit for recent onset of tiredness and frequent urination

BACKGROUND

- Four months ago you saw this patient in clinic for a check-up. He had no complaints. You performed a complete history and physical examination.
- His FMH was significant for diabetes and high cholesterol.
- At the last visit, you ordered electrolytes and cholesterol and told him to make a follow-up appointment to review his labs 2 weeks later. He cancelled the appointment.
- As you review his EMR before the visit you notice his sugar was 190 on the lab work you ordered 4 months ago. There is nothing in the record to suggest that you responded to this abnormality.
- Today he presents complaining of fatigue, excessive urination, and thirst.
- His finger stick is 250 and urine dip has glucose.

YOUR ROLE

Resident on ambulatory care rotation

YOUR TASKS

- Explain the follow-up error
- Explore the patient's current problem
- Develop a plan
- DO NOT CONDUCT A PHYSICAL EXAM

SP instructions: MEDICAL ERROR DISCLOSURE

SCENARIO

Your name is John McCoy. You are 42 years old and single. You are a jazz pianist but have been waiting in order to make ends meet.

Four months ago you came to the clinic for the first time. You realized that you had not been to a doctor for a while and should have a check-up. Your mom has diabetes and takes tons of medications and your father has high cholesterol and is crazy about what he eats. While you keep a pretty healthy life style in terms of diet and exercise and consider yourself too young to have problems, you thought your family history might put you at risk so you decided to get checked out.

You liked the doctor you saw the last time you were here. You felt (s)he listened and took your concerns seriously. (S)he ordered tests to check your sugar and cholesterol. You got your blood drawn fasting (as the doctor requested) and made a follow-up appointment. Unfortunately you had to cancel it at the last minute because of an unexpected music gig (these don't come across as often as you'd like). When you called to cancel the computer system was down and the receptionist said that you would have to call back. When you called again later you got a busy signal and gave up trying to get through. No one from the clinic called you back to reschedule, so you figured that the results must have been fine anyway.

About 2 weeks ago you started to feel really exhausted. You noticed that you were constantly thirsty and going to the bathroom a lot. You started to keep a plastic liter bottle of water with you at all times and needing to refill it frequently. You are urinating constantly, at high volume but without any associated pain. It seems like all of your clothes are little loose and you wonder whether you've also lost a few pounds (you are of medium build, your weight is usually steady).

Finally you missed several days of work because the constant bathroom runs were really disruptive to your work in the restaurant. You had someone cover for you at your job but you were afraid that you would not get your day shift back. Yesterday, you decided to work anyway even though you seem to be running to the bathroom every 10 min. By the end of the day you were totally exhausted and anxious.

For the last 4 days you have been calling the clinic daily trying to make an appointment with the same physician you saw the last time. Finally, today, the doctor is able to see you. You are feeling exhausted, a little worried about what is wrong with you, and frustrated with the clinic appointment system. Today you've already had to wait more than an hour before getting to see the doctor. You are expected at your job shortly.

HISTORY OF PRESENT ILLNESS	Chief complaint:	Tiredness, frequent urination.
	Where	General exhaustion.
	When	Problem started about 2 weeks ago, you are going to the bathroom every 10 min, waking frequently at night.
	Quality	Exhausted due to lack of sleep. No pain on urination.
	Quantity	High volume urination.
	Aggravating/ allevia-ting factors	None.
	Associated symptoms	Increased thirst, possible weight loss, no fever.
	Beliefs	Fear it may be diabetes like your mother has.

CURRENT LIFE SITUATION

You moved to New York City when you were 20 and have been living with a roommate in the East Village for the last 10 years. You have never been married and have no children but you have had a number of steady girlfriends and are usually in a relationship. Your parents live in Ohio, as does your 2-year younger brother, who is married.

You work as a waiter at the Café Wha and intermittently play jazz piano with various local groups. You are still hoping to make it as a pianist, but it hasn't worked out that well so far. Your financial situation is slightly unstable which can put you on edge at times.

Over the last few months nothing much has changed in your life. You job has been as stressful as always. No change in your diet or exercise either. You have recently started to become worried that you might have diabetes.

PERSONALITY

You tend to be a little dramatic. When you are happy, you are very upbeat and when you are upset, you can get quite angry, raising your voice (although not shouting or swearing).

PAST MEDICAL HISTORY

Common childhood diseases and colds—otherwise unremarkable

No past surgical or psychiatric history

FAMILY MEDICAL HISTORY

Your mother has had diabetes for about 15 years (you think she was diagnosed at age 45). You know that it has been getting worse and fear that she does not take great care of herself.

You father has high cholesterol and obsessed with his health. He is always on a special diet and cooks all his own food. In your opinion, your parents have a strange relationship but it seems to work for them.

MEDICATIONS None

ALLERGIES None

SOCIAL HISTORY

You do not smoke and do not use recreational drugs. You drink alcohol at least three times per week, usually having 2–3 drinks each time.

You are sexually active (using condoms for protection) with a girlfriend whom you have had for the past 6 months.

Normally, you eat and sleeping well (when work allows) and stay active by going to the gym occasionally. Of course your restaurant job also keeps you moving constantly.

ENCOUNTER BEGINNING

When the resident enters the room, you are sitting in a chair in the exam room talking to a waiter colleague on a cell phone, trying to get someone to cover for you as you may be late for work today since you are still at the doctor's office. You are upset, interrupting the person on the other end of the phone line, and end the conversation about 20 s after the resident enters the room. When you hang up, you are still upset about having to miss work although you are glad to finally see the physician again. You express some frustration about not getting an appointment sooner, waiting so long in the waiting room which results in more work problems, and never hearing back about the test results.

If asked in an open-ended way why you are here, state: "I'm feeling really awful, I am peeing all the time and I never found out what my blood tests showed."

Provide details about your current state as indicated above.

How have you been before problem started? – "Fine, I guess. I have been busy at work and trying to get as many music gigs as I can. Maybe I was a little thirsty. I think I lost a few pounds, but who pays attention. I don't really keep regular hours."

MIDDLE   **If/when you are told a mistake was made** (i.e., the fasting blood tests you did 4 months ago showed you had diabetes, all other labs were normal), regardless of where it occurs in the interview, take a moment to let it set in and then respond with anger. Raise your voice (but don't shout), look the resident straight in the eye and state: "So I had diabetes 4 months ago? Why didn't anyone call me? Is this what is going on now?" and: "Could we have avoided all this? What's going on here? I had to miss days of work because of this! Will there be any long-term damage because you did not catch this earlier? You mean I could have been dying and no one would have told me my blood sugar was high unless I came here. Aren't there systems to contact patients with abnormal tests? I assumed no news was good news."

When you realize the **long-term damage will be nil or minimal**, you become a little less agitated but state in a frustrated way: "Why did this happen? What if this was something really serious? I mean, my God, does this happen here all the time? There is something wrong with the system here!"

If the resident remains **apologetic and non-confrontational**, you calm down a little and ask: "Well, when can I go back to work? How am I going to get better?"

If the resident acknowledges that a mistake was made, but then becomes **defensive, does not empathize** or say (s)he is sorry or makes up a bizarre story, get more upset: "I mean, me missing work today would have been totally unnecessary right? If you guys actually did your job, I wouldn't have had to get so sick. I knew I shouldn't have come to this clinic." If the resident blames you for not rescheduling explain that when you called to cancel the computer system was down and no one contacted you when it was up again. Thus you surmised that it was not so important.

Ongoing: If the resident is empathic/truthful/straightforward, become more and more calm. If the resident is defensive or evasive become more and more upset/angry.

END (2 min warning)   **Regardless of resident's reactions**, calm down a bit and stop additional questions about how this happened to allow the interviewer close down the encounter. State: "Well, so I have diabetes. Now what?"

If the resident is acting appropriately you calm down in response to the effective interventions. If the resident acted inappropriately, mention that you intend to take up the problem with someone else. Cross your arms and avoid eye contact but stop making angry comments.

The following is an SP checklist for the "Medical Error Disclosure" case included in Appendix F, above.

Medical Error Disclosure

Resident ID #		SP Name:

COMMUNICATION

Information gathering	Not done	Partially done	Well done	*Comments*
Elicited your responses using appropriate questions: • No leading questions • Only 1 question at a time	Impeded story by asking leading/judgmental questions AND more than one question at a time	Used leading/judgmental questions OR asked more than one question at a time	Asked questions one at a time without leading patient in their responses	
Clarified information by repeating to make sure he/she understood you on an ongoing basis	Did not clarify (did not repeat back to you the information you provided)	Repeated information you provided but did not give you a chance to indicate if accurate	Repeated information and directly invited you to indicate whether accurate	
Allowed you to talk *without interrupting*	Interrupted	Did not interrupt directly BUT cut responses short by not giving enough time	Did not interrupt AND allowed time to express thoughts fully	
Relationship development	Not done	Partially done	Well done	*Comments*
Communicated concern or intention to help	Did not communicate intention to help/concern via words or actions	Words OR actions conveyed intention to help/concern	Actions AND words conveyed intention to help/concern	
Nonverbal behavior enriched communication (e.g., eye contact, posture)	Nonverbal behavior was negative OR interfered with communication	Nonverbal behavior demonstrated attentiveness	Nonverbal behavior facilitated effective communication	
Acknowledged emotions/ feelings appropriately	DID NOT acknowledge emotions/feelings	Acknowledged emotions/ feelings	Acknowledged and responded to emotions/feelings in ways that made you feel better	
Was *accepting/ nonjudgmental*	Made judgmental comments OR facial expressions	Did not express judgment but did not demonstrate respect	Made comments and expressions that demonstrated respect	

Used words you understood and/or explained *jargon*	Consistently used jargon WITHOUT further explanation	Sometimes used jargon AND did not explain it	Explained jargon when used OR avoided jargon completely	
Patient education and counseling	**Not done**	**Partially done**	**Well done**	*Comments*
Asked questions to see what you understood (check your understanding)	Did not check for understanding	Asked if patient had any questions BUT did not check for understanding	Assessed understanding by checking in throughout the encounter	
Provided *clear explanations*/information	Gave confusing OR no explanations which made it impossible to understand information	Information was somewhat clear BUT still led to some difficulty in understanding	Provided small bits of information at a time AND summarized to ensure understanding	
Collaborated with you in identifying possible next steps/plan	Told patient next steps/plan	Told patient next steps THEN asked patient's views	Told patient options, THEN mutually developed a plan of action	

CASE-SPECIFIC SKILLS

Delivering bad news	**Not done**	**Partially done**	**Well done**	*Comments*
Prepared you to receive the news: • Entered room prepared to deliver news • Ensured sufficient time and privacy	Entered room in a manner unfitting the news AND physically situated self far away	Entered room in a manner unfitting the news OR physically situated him/ herself far from you	Entered room in a manner befitting the news AND physically situated him/herself close to you	
Gave a *warning shot* (e.g., "I have some bad news for you…")	No warning shot	Attempted to deliver warning shot, BUT did so inappropriately (did not pause for your assent OR warning shot too long)	Gave you a well-timed warning shot	
Gave you *opportunity to respond*: • Remained sensitive to your venting of shock, anger, disbelief, accusations • Attended to your emotions before moving on	Responded inappropriately to your emotional reaction (no opportunity to vent, cut you off, became defensive)	Allowed you to emotionally respond (vent) BUT did not address/acknowledge response before moving on	Allowed you to express your feelings, fully giving you the feeling you were being listened to before moving on	
Directly asked what you are feeling: "What are you thinking/feeling?"	Did not ask specifically "What are you thinking/ feeling?"	Acknowledged your feelings (e.g., "I see that you are upset…") BUT did not ask you to name your emotions	Specifically asked you "What are you thinking/feeling?"	
Managing a difficult situation	**Not done**	**Partially done**	**Well done**	*Comments*
Avoided *assigning blame*	Became defensive/ argumentative AND assigned blame to a person/department	Became defensive/ argumentative OR assigned blame to a person/department	Remained calm AND did not mention blame someone else	
Maintained professionalism by *controlling emotions*	Unable to control emotions, became dismissive, defensive, or condescending	Attempted to control emotions (e.g. only somewhat dismissive, defensive, or condescending)	Maintained high level of professionalism, no defensiveness, anger, frustration	

Disclosure and accountability	Not done	Partially done	Well done	*Comments*
Disclosed error • Direct (used the words "error" or "mistake") • Prompt disclosure	Did not directly disclose the error (there was a "problem") NOR was the explanation upfront	Did not directly disclose the error (there was a "problem") OR directly disclosed late in the interview	Directly disclosed the error upfront	
Personally *apologized* for the error ("I am sorry that this happened")	Did not apologize for error NOR for the inconvenience it caused you	Apologized for the error OR for the inconvenience it caused you	Apologized for the error AND for the inconvenience it caused you	
Shared the *cause of the error* (i.e., explained issues with system)	Did not acknowledge issues with system	Acknowledged issue with system BUT was dismissive/condescending	Acknowledged issue with system AND was genuine in addressing it	
Took *responsibility* for situation	Took no personal responsibility for your present situation (e.g., assigns your problem to other person/department)	Took a general responsibility as part of the department for your present situation	Took a personal responsibility for your situation ("I will…")	
Identified future *preventive strategies* to prevent situation from happening again	Did not address how situation would be prevented in future	Made general suggestion for improvement (e.g., "We'll look into it," "I'll make a note of it to my Attending")	Offered specific strategies for potential improvement of system	

PATIENT SATISFACTION

The doctor (resident)….	Not done	Partially done	Well done	*Comments*
Fully explored my *experience of the problem* (concerns, symptoms, functions, feelings, ideas)	Did not explore	Explored some aspects of my experience but not all	Fully explored major aspects of my experience	
Explored my *expectations about visit* (problem, solution)	Did not explore	Partially explored my expectations	Fully explored my expectations	
Took a *personal interest* in me; treated me as a *person*	Did not see me as a person	Viewed me as a person, but did not take personal interest	Took an active personal interest in me	
Gave me *enough information*	I was not given any where close to enough information	I was given some information but I still had questions	I was given all the information I wanted/needed	

The following form (details tailored to the "Medical Error Disclosure" case [Appendix F]) is intended to assist faculty observers in evaluating OSCE participant (resident, in this case) performance.

COMMUNICATION

	Does not meet expectations	Meets expectations	Exceeds expectations	Comments
Information gathering	1. Elicited patient responses using appropriate questions (no leading questions, only 1 question at a time) 2. Clarified information by repeating to make sure he/she understood patient on an ongoing basis 3. Allowed patient to talk without interrupting			

	Does not meet expectations	Meets expectations	Exceeds expectations	Comments
Relationship development	1. Communicated concern or intention to help 2. Nonverbal behavior enriched communication (eye contact, posture) 3. Acknowledged emotions/feelings appropriately 4. Was accepting/nonjudgmental 5. Used words patient understood and/or explained jargon			

	Does not meet expectations	Meets expectations	Exceeds expectations	Comments
Patient education and counseling	1. Asked questions to see what patient understood (checked for understanding) 2. Provided clear explanations/information 3. Collaborated with patient in identifying possible next steps/plan			

CASE-SPECIFIC SKILLS

	Does not meet expectations	Meets expectations	Exceeds expectations	Comments
Disclosing error	1. Used "breaking bad news format", i.e., prepared patient, gave warning shot, was unambiguous in delivery, gave patient an opportunity to respond 2. Was prompt and direct with disclosure ("I made a mistake"), personally apologized, and took responsibility for next steps 3. Shared cause of error, and let patient know what would be done to prevent error from happening again			

S. Zabar et al. (eds.), *Objective Structured Clinical Examinations*,
DOI 10.1007/978-1-4614-3749-9, © Springer Science+Business Media New York 2013

Managing a difficult situation	**Does not meet expectations**	**Meets expectations**	**Exceeds expectations**	*Comments*
	1. Maintained professional composure and controlled emotions 2. Avoided assigning blame—to someone else within "the system" or to the patient			

Overall, how would you rate this resident in each of the following areas....?

	Unacceptable	Does not meet expectations	Meets expectations	Above expectations	Outstanding
Communication skills	1	2	3	4	5
Comments:					
Medical knowledge	1	2	3	4	5
Comments:					
Professionalism	1	2	3	4	5
Comments:					

Additional Comments:

Appendix I
OSCE Case/Station Development

Template for developing materials for an OSCE station (Station Overview, Participant Instructions, SP Instructions).

Station overview: CASE/STATION NAME

DEVELOPMENT DATE	
STATION DEVELOPER(S) (contact information)	
LEARNERS (intended and potential)	
OBJECTIVES	To test learners' ability to: 1. 2. 3. 4.
LOGISTICS	Personnel: Forms: <ul><li>Resident instructions</li><li>SP instructions</li><li>SP rating form</li><li>Faculty rating form</li></ul> Room requirements/resources:

S. Zabar et al. (eds.), *Objective Structured Clinical Examinations*,
DOI 10.1007/978-1-4614-3749-9, © Springer Science+Business Media New York 2013

Participant instructions: CASE/STATION NAME

PATIENT INFORMATION	Name: Age: Marital status: Occupation:
REASON FOR ENCOUNTER **BACKGROUND**	• • • • •
YOUR ROLE **YOUR TASKS**	• • • (indicate if a physical exam is expected)

SP instructions: CASE/STATION NAME

SCENARIO	Your name is … (how did the current encounter come about?)	
HISTORY OF PRESENT ILLNESS	Chief complaint:	(reason for visit)
	Where	(location and radiation of symptom)
	When	(when it began, fluctuation over time, duration)
	Quality	(what it feels like)
	Quantity	(intensity, extent, degree of disability)
	Aggravating/alleviating factors	(what makes it better/worse)
	Associated symptoms	(other manifestations)
	Beliefs	(what does the patient think is wrong)
CURRENT LIFE SITUATION	(where does patient live/work, …)	
PERSONALITY	(key emotional tone and approach to responses)	
PAST MEDICAL HISTORY	(past illnesses including surgical or psychiatric conditions)	
FAMILY MEDICAL HISTORY	(past medical, surgical, and/or psychiatric conditions relevant for the case)	
MEDICATIONS	(list with quantity if relevant)	
ALLERGIES	(list)	
SOCIAL HISTORY	(e.g., smoking, drugs, alcohol, diet, exercise)	
ENCOUNTER BEGINNING	(what SP should do at the beginning of the encounter, opening statement)	
MIDDLE	(how the SP should respond with information and emotionally given various learner approaches)	
END (2 min warning)	(how the SP should allow the learner to close the encounter)	
PHYSICAL EXAM	(how the SP should react to relevant physical exam maneuvers, what the participant will be looking for)	

The following checklist template can be adapted for any case by adding case-specific items and anchors and removing any non-applicable sections (e.g., physical exam).

| [place participant ID here] | Case name: _____ |
| | SP Name: |

COMMUNICATION

Information gathering	Not done	Partially done	Well done	Comments
Elicited your responses using appropriate questions: • No leading questions • Only 1 question at a time	Impeded story by asking leading/judgmental questions AND more than one question at a time	Used leading/judgmental questions OR asked more than one question at a time	Asked questions one at a time without leading patient in their responses	
Clarified information by repeating to make sure he/she understood you on an ongoing basis	Did not clarify (did not repeat back to you the information you provided)	Repeated information you provided but did not give you a chance to indicate if accurate	Repeated information and directly invited you to indicate whether accurate	
Allowed you to talk *without interrupting*	Interrupted	Did not interrupt directly BUT cut responses short by not giving enough time	Did not interrupt AND allowed time to express thoughts fully	
Relationship development	Not done	Partially done	Well done	Comments
Communicated concern or intention to help	Did not communicate intention to help/concern via words or actions	Words OR actions conveyed intention to help/concern	Actions AND words conveyed intention to help/concern	
Nonverbal behavior enriched communication (e.g., eye contact, posture)	Nonverbal behavior was negative OR interfered with communication	Nonverbal behavior demonstrated attentiveness	Nonverbal behavior facilitated effective communication	
Acknowledged emotions/feelings appropriately	DID NOT acknowledge emotions/feelings	Acknowledged emotions/feelings	Acknowledged and responded to emotions/feelings in ways that made you feel better	

Was *accepting/ nonjudgmental*	Made judgmental comments OR facial expressions	Did not express judgment but did not demonstrate respect	Made comments and expressions that demonstrated respect	
Used words you understood and/or explained *jargon*	Consistently used jargon WITHOUT further explanation	Sometimes used jargon AND did not explain it	Explained jargon when used OR avoided jargon completely	
Patient education and counseling	**Not done**	**Partially done**	**Well done**	*Comments*
Asked questions to see what you understood (check your understanding)	Did not check for understanding	Asked if patient had any questions BUT did not check for understanding	Assessed understanding by checking in throughout the encounter	
Provided *clear explanations*/information	Gave confusing OR no explanations which made it impossible to understand information	Information was somewhat clear BUT still led to some difficulty in understanding	Provided small bits of information at a time AND summarized to ensure understanding	
Collaborated with you in identifying possible next steps/plan	Told patient next steps/ plan	Told patient next steps THEN asked patient's views	Told patient options, THEN mutually developed a plan of action	

CASE-SPECIFIC SKILLS

*Competency:*_____	**Not done**	**Partially done**	**Well done**	*Comments*
1.				
2.				
3.				
*Competency:*_____	**Not done**	**Partially done**	**Well done**	*Comments*
1.				
2.				
3.				
*Competency:*_____	**Not done**	**Partially done**	**Well done**	*Comments*
1.				
2.				
3.				

PHYSICAL EXAM

*Competency:*_____	**Not done**	**Partially done**	**Well done**	*Comments*
1.				
2.				
*Competency:*_____	**Not done**	**Partially done**	**Well done**	*Comments*
1.				
2.				

PATIENT SATISFACTION

The doctor (resident)….	Not done	Partially done	Well done	Comments
Fully explored my *experience of the problem* (concerns, symptoms, functions, feelings, ideas)	Did not explore	Explored some aspects of my experience but not all	Fully explored major aspects of my experience	
Explored my *expectations about visit* (problem, solution)	Did not explore	Partially explored my expectations	Fully explored my expectations	
Took a *personal interest* in me; treated me as a *person*	Did not see me as a person	Viewed me as a person, but did not take personal interest	Took an active personal interest in me	
Gave me *enough information*	I was not given any where close to enough information	I was given some information but I still had questions	I was given all the information I wanted/ needed	

PATIENT ACTIVATION

This encounter….	Not done	Partially done	Well done	Comments
This encounter helped me to *understand the nature and causes* of my problem	Did not help me understand	Helped me understand some things but not everything	Helped me fully understand what happened	
After the encounter, I *knew and understood the different medical treatment options available*	I did not find out about treatment options	I found out about some of the treatment options	I found out about all of the relevant treatment options	
This visit made me feel *confident I can keep my problem interfering* too much with my life	Did not affect my confidence	Helped me feel more confident that I could keep my health problem from interfering with life	Helped me feel very confident that I could keep my health problem from interfering with life	
Because of this encounter, *I am confident I can figure out solutions if something new* comes up	Did not affect my confidence	Helped me feel somewhat confident that I could deal with new issues	Helped me feel quite confident that I could deal with new issues	

Would you recommend this doctor to a friend or family member for his/her….?

COMMUNICATION SKILLS:	Not recommend	Recommend with reservations	Recommend	Highly recommend
MEDICAL COMPETENCE:	Not recommend	Recommend with reservations	Recommend	Highly recommend

Overall, how would you rate this doctor's professionalism?

	Not at all professional	Somewhat professional	Professional	Very professional
Professionalism	*Most* of the following • Disrespectful • Not compassionate • Not accountable • Not sensitive/ responsive to my needs/situation	*A few* of the following • Disrespectful • Not compassionate • Not accountable • Not sensitive/ responsive to my needs/situation	*3* of the following • Respectful • Compassionate • Accountable • Sensitive/responsive to my needs/situation	*All* of the following • Respectful • Compassionate • Accountable • Sensitive/responsive to my needs/situation

SPECIFIC (<1 min) FEEDBACK:

COMMENTS (additional remarks, factors affecting your score, impressions)

Appendix K
Survey: Participant Evaluation of OSCE Experience

(designed for a residency OSCE; PGY = post-graduate year)

Please indicate your response to each of the three questions listed in the columns:

Station #	Case	How much *exposure* have you had to similar cases?			How *difficult* was this case for you?			How much did you *learn* from doing this case?			How would you rate your *overall performance* in this case?				What did you think was *the point* of this case?
		None	Some	A lot	Too easy	Just right	Too hard	Nothing	Some	A lot	Poor	Fair	Good	Excellent	
1		☐	☐	☐	☐	☐	☐	☐	☐	☐	☐	☐	☐	☐	
2		☐	☐	☐	☐	☐	☐	☐	☐	☐	☐	☐	☐	☐	
3		☐	☐	☐	☐	☐	☐	☐	☐	☐	☐	☐	☐	☐	
4		☐	☐	☐	☐	☐	☐	☐	☐	☐	☐	☐	☐	☐	
5		☐	☐	☐	☐	☐	☐	☐	☐	☐	☐	☐	☐	☐	
6		☐	☐	☐	☐	☐	☐	☐	☐	☐	☐	☐	☐	☐	
7		☐	☐	☐	☐	☐	☐	☐	☐	☐	☐	☐	☐	☐	
8		☐	☐	☐	☐	☐	☐	☐	☐	☐	☐	☐	☐	☐	
9		☐	☐	☐	☐	☐	☐	☐	☐	☐	☐	☐	☐	☐	
10		☐	☐	☐	☐	☐	☐	☐	☐	☐	☐	☐	☐	☐	

Please indicate how much you agree or disagree with each of the items below:

	In general this OSCE…..	Strongly DISAGREE	Somewhat DISAGREE	Somewhat AGREE	Strongly AGREE
1	Helped me identify my strengths and weaknesses	☐	☐	☐	☐
2	Stimulated me so that I'll go and learn more about some of the topics covered	☐	☐	☐	☐
3	Taught me something new	☐	☐	☐	☐
4	Provided me with valuable feedback	☐	☐	☐	☐
5	Was a lot like real-life clinical encounters	☐	☐	☐	☐
6	Evaluated my skills fairly	☐	☐	☐	☐
7	Was enjoyable	☐	☐	☐	☐
8	Provided a good cross section of general medicine	☐	☐	☐	☐
9	Was an experience I would like to have again	☐	☐	☐	☐

FOR PGY2s and PGY3s ONLY
If you've completed this OSCE before…

S. Zabar et al. (eds.), *Objective Structured Clinical Examinations*,
DOI 10.1007/978-1-4614-3749-9, © Springer Science+Business Media New York 2013

					Comments
How well did you do on this OSCE compared with the previous one(s)?	I Did Much Worse on this OSCE ☐	About the Same ☐	I Did Much Better on this OSCE ☐	*NOT APPLICABLE* ☐	

We welcome any comments, feedback, suggestions—about the OSCE, the Standardized Patients, the whole process…

Appendix L
Survey: Faculty Evaluation of OSCE Experience

(designed for General Internal Medicine faculty observers in a residency OSCE)

Please indicate your response to each of the three questions listed in the columns:

Case #	Case	How difficult was this case for the residents?			How much will residents learn from this case?			How well did the SP play this case?			Overall, how well did the residents (as a group) perform in this case?				What was most surprising about the residents' performance?
		Too easy	Just right	Too Hard	Nothing	Some	A lot	Not well	O.K.	Very well	Poor	Fair	Good	Excellent	
		☐	☐	☐	☐	☐	☐	☐	☐	☐	☐	☐	☐	☐	
		☐	☐	☐	☐	☐	☐	☐	☐	☐	☐	☐	☐	☐	

Please indicate how much you agree or disagree with each of the items below:

In general this OSCE…..	Strongly DISAGREE	Somewhat DISAGREE	Somewhat AGREE	Strongly AGREE
1 Helped residents identify their strengths and weaknesses	☐	☐	☐	☐
2 Will stimulated residents to learn more about some of the topics covered	☐	☐	☐	☐
3 Taught residents something new	☐	☐	☐	☐
4 Provided residents with valuable feedback	☐	☐	☐	☐
5 Provided me with new information about residents' performance level	☐	☐	☐	☐
6 Gave me some new ideas for teaching	☐	☐	☐	☐
7 Was a lot like real-life clinical encounters	☐	☐	☐	☐
8 Evaluated residents' skills fairly	☐	☐	☐	☐
9 Was enjoyable	☐	☐	☐	☐
10 Provided a good cross section of general medicine	☐	☐	☐	☐
11 Was an experience I, as faculty, would like to have again	☐	☐	☐	☐

We welcome comments, feedback, suggestions—about the OSCE, the rating form, the SPs, the whole process….

Comments:

S. Zabar et al. (eds.), *Objective Structured Clinical Examinations*,
DOI 10.1007/978-1-4614-3749-9, © Springer Science+Business Media New York 2013

STANDARDIZED PATIENT EVALUATION OF THE OSCE EXPERIENCE

Please indicate your response to each of the three questions listed in the columns:

Case #	Case	How difficult was this case for the participants?			How much will participants learn from this case?			Overall, how well did the participants (as a group) perform in this case?				What was most surprising about the participants' performance?
		Too easy	Just right	Too hard	Nothing	Some	A lot	Poor	Fair	Good	Excellent	
		☐	☐	☐	☐	☐	☐	☐	☐	☐	☐	

Were there any consistent problems with using the checklist? Items that didn't seem to work? Aspects of the participants' performance that weren't reflected?

Was there anything about your character that was didn't work? Were there any questions asked that you felt unprepared for?

Did any of the participants say or do anything that you felt unprepared to handle?

How did it go giving feedback? Any problems? Any highlights? Suggestions for improvement?

Is there anything that we can do to better prepare you? (playing the case, rating performance, giving feedback, staying alert?)

Appendix N
Sample USP Case

Included below are SP instructions for the "Trouble Breathing/Asthma" USP case, designed to evaluate resident physician performance and the clinical microsystem in a primary care outpatient setting. Highlighted case details are varied each visit to minimize USP detectability.

SP Instructions: TROUBLE BREATHING/ASTHMA

SCENARIO	You are a 23–26-year-old female with a history of asthma. You've been living in New York City a little over a year
	You came into the clinic today because your asthma has been much worse in the last week. This past week you've been up a lot at night because of trouble breathing and twice had to use your inhaler 3 times in one night. You knew this was bad, that you shouldn't be using it so much
	You've had asthma since you were a little kid, but it's never been that bad. Usually it only affected you when you had a cold, and it never stopped you from doing anything. When you had a cold, you would cough a lot, but it would get better with an inhaler
	When you moved from Baltimore last winter, your asthma started getting much worse. Over the summer it got better, but this winter it's been bad again. If asked if you think the weather is the reason for your increased asthma, you shrug it off with "I don't know, I just know it's gotten worse"
	You never went to the ER until last winter when you had a bad attack. *This winter* you've been to the ER (New York Downtown Hospital) a total of 3 times over the past winter
	For the past few months you have been experiencing a very bad cough (hacking, no phlegm). You also have wheezing, shortness of breath (dyspnea), and chest tightness. This happens especially at night, when you go out into the cold or when you walk upstairs
	Last week you had a cold (stuffy, runny nose but no fever) that got better on its own. However, over the last few days your breathing has been much worse. Other ways to describe asthma: "chest tightness—when I take a deep breath, my chest hits a wall half way through what would be a normal breath"
	You use an albuterol inhaler which helps your symptoms and another inhaler (it is kind of coral colored—you don't remember the name of it [Flovent]) that you are supposed to take every day (actually, if specifically asked, you are supposed to take it twice daily, once in the morning, once at night) but stopped using after 2 days because "it doesn't do anything."
	You were prescribed the coral-colored inhaler at the ER when your asthma first got really bad when you moved to NYC last winter. If asked if you still have it, you do—it's somewhere in your bathroom. *You are not aware that the Flovent is a preventive medication*
	This winter, you've found yourself having to use the albuterol inhaler more than usual (until last year you only used it for rare attacks), about three times a week. Over the past month, you started using the inhaler once or twice a day. It seems like you need to use the inhaler "every time you do anything," including walking up the subway steps, and light housework. Last week, things got even worse and you needed the inhaler 3 times in one night on 2 different nights. You don't really like taking the albuterol because even though it helps you breathe better, it makes you anxious and jittery

S. Zabar et al. (eds.), *Objective Structured Clinical Examinations*,
DOI 10.1007/978-1-4614-3749-9, © Springer Science+Business Media New York 2013

HISTORY OF PRESENT ILLNESS	Chief complaint:	Difficulty breathing and asthma attacks
	Where	General respiratory
	When	Problem has been getting increasingly worse in past 3 months
	Quality	Debilitating
	Quantity	3 attacks in one night at its worst
	Aggravating/alleviating factors	Aggravating: cold, nighttime, activity, poor air quality; Alleviating (temporary): albuterol inhaler
	Associated symptoms	Hacking cough, wheezing, shortness of breath, low energy
	Beliefs	You don't like to consider yourself "sick," and prefer not to take medications or see a doctor at all. However, your worry about your job makes you feel like you have to get this "taken care of"
		You have not had a regular doctor since moving from home
CURRENT LIFE SITUATION	You live with your boyfriend from home in an apartment in Manhattan (Stuyvesant Town) that belongs to your grandmother, who can no longer live on her own and is now living with your family back in Baltimore. You lived at home through college and moved to NYC with your boyfriend after graduation	
	Your mom is pretty high-strung and she is getting upset that you are sick all the time. You talk on the phone a lot and she is worried you are missing too much work	
	You work in a restaurant/retail store. You are worried about getting fired because you were home sick a few times over the winter, starting when the weather got cold	
PERSONALITY	You are a quiet and friendly person but a bit intimidated by health care providers	
PAST MEDICAL HISTORY	Besides your asthma, you've had no medical problems. Never hospitalized	
	You have had all your vaccinations (your mother has the "little yellow book" where these are written down)	
FAMILY MEDICAL HISTORY	Your parents have no medical problems. You are not aware of anyone else in your family having asthma	
MEDICATIONS	Regular albuterol inhaler, plus "coral-colored" inhaler prescribed at the ER. No previous medications prescribed for Asthma	
	You have been on birth control (Yaz) for 4 years	
ALLERGIES	You don't have any allergies to medicines. Cats usually bother your asthma, you've never had pets. Cigarette smoke also makes you cough	
SOCIAL HISTORY	Sexual history	You've been with your current boyfriend since you were seniors in high school. You had 2 sexual partners before him and you always use condoms
	Smoking	You've never smoked, and no one at home or at work smokes
	Alcohol/Drugs	Occasionally you have a beer. No drugs
	Nutrition	You eat mostly healthy food. No recent weight gain
	Exercise	No exercise besides being on your feet all day at work
INTERVIEW CHALLENGES FOR RESIDENT	• Take a focused history concerning asthma symptoms now and over the past year • Explore patient's motivation for taking medications (stop coughing, keep up at work, stop going to ER) • Recommend/counsel on using medications regularly and keeping doctor's appointments	
ENCOUNTER BEGINNING	State how you've been feeling the last few days. If asked about how the problem has been in the past, explain the worsening of the condition this and last winter and how you've been to the ER a few times	
MIDDLE	If the resident does not ask about how your asthma is affecting you relate that you are missing a lot of work and sleeping pretty poorly which makes it hard to have any energy. If asked about this, state you're actually pretty worried	
	If asked about taking medications regularly (not just "when you need them"), you state that you are a little reluctant to do so. You actually don't think the coral-colored inhaler really works since you didn't feel anything when you used it. You are worried about using an inhaler in front of your boss or coworkers because you feel like they will think you are weak and sickly, but it is also pretty embarrassing that you can't run up the stairs without huffing and puffing. You have never seen anyone else use an asthma pump. Sometimes you are not sure whether you are using the pump correctly (take out your pump at that time to give the physician an opportunity to let you demonstrate how you do it). (We will show you how to do it a little wrong)	
	If medications are explained and your understanding of them is checked, state that you are willing to take the 2 daily preventive pumps of Flovent. You are motivated to get better because you feel horrible and hate going to the ER. You want to be "normal." You would be willing to see a doctor regularly if you didn't have to miss work	
	If the resident does not come up with a follow-up plan or medication plan, say something like "maybe I'm on the wrong medications…"	
END	You're pleased about having received more information about your problem. You are an intelligent person and no one had ever explained to you before that the two asthma meds worked in different ways. You are happy about the prospect of getting your asthma under control	

The following resident performance and clinical microsystem checklist ("Trouble Breathing/Asthma" case) is completed by the SP after the USP encounter.

Date:	
MD Name:	

Asthma

SP Name: _____

Clinic Team _____

When did you arrive at your appointed clinic area?	_____:_____	am/pm
When did your visit with the resident begin?	_____:_____	am/pm
When did your visit end?	_____:_____	am/pm

Comments

The primary care associate...			*Comments*	
1st PCA	**2nd PCA** (if applicable)		**1st PCA**	**2nd PCA**
☐	☐	Greeted me within a reasonable time frame		
☐	☐	Introduced self		
☐	☐	Wore a visible name tag		
☐	☐	Asked me my name		
☐	☐	Asked me my date of birth		
☐	☐	Washed hands before touching me		
☐	☐	Measured my height		
☐	☐	Took my blood pressure		
☐	☐	Weighed me		
☐	☐	Screened for depression using the PHQ-2		
Acknowledged/apologized for any delays	**1st PCA**	☐ No	☐ Yes	☐ NA (No Delays)
	2nd PCA	☐ No	☐ Yes	☐ NA (No Delays)
Was friendly and/or professional	**1st PCA**	☐ Rude	☐ Professional	☐ Friendly
	2nd PCA	☐ Rude	☐ Professional	☐ Friendly
Took care to explain things to me	**1st PCA**	☐ No Explaining	☐ Some Explaining	☐ Fully Explained
	2nd PCA	☐ No Explaining	☐ Some Explaining	☐ Fully Explained
Overall, were you satisfied overall with the way the PCAs treated you?		☐ Not Satisfied	☐ Somewhat Satisfied	☐ Very Satisfied
Comments:				

Experience with clinic			
It was easy to navigate through the system	☐ Not So Easy	☐ Relatively Easy	☐ Very Easy
The *team* to which I was assigned functioned well	☐ Problems	☐ Functioned O.K.	☐ Functioned Well
Overall, I was treated professionally by non-MD staff	☐ Not At All	☐ Somewhat Professional	☐ Very Professional
Comments:			

COMMUNICATION SKILLS

Information gathering	Not done	Partially done	Well done	Comments
Elicited your responses using appropriate questions	Asked leading questions AND more than one question at a time	Used leading questions OR asked more than one question at a time	Asked questions one at a time without leading you in your response	
Managed the narrative flow of your story	Not able to elicit your story because questions are not organized logically	Elicited main elements of story, but illogical order of questions disrupted flow	Elicited full story by asking questions that facilitated natural flow of story	
Clarified information throughout by repeating to make sure understood you	Did not clarify (did not repeat back to you the information you provided)	Repeated info you provided but did not give you a chance to indicate accuracy	Repeated info and directly invited you to indicate accuracy	
Allowed you to talk without interrupting	Interrupted	Did not interrupt BUT cut responses short, not enough time	Did not interrupt; allowed to express thoughts fully	

Relationship development	Not done	Partially done	Well done	Comments
Communicated concern or intention to help	Did not communicate intention to help/concern	Words OR actions conveyed intention to help/concern	Actions AND words conveyed intention to help/concern	
Nonverbal behavior enriched communication (e.g., eye contact, posture)	Nonverbal behavior was negative OR interfered with communication	Nonverbal behavior demonstrated attentiveness	Nonverbal behavior facilitated effective communication	
Acknowledged emotions/feelings appropriately	DID NOT acknowledge emotions/feelings	Acknowledged emotions/feelings	Acknowledged and responded in ways that made you feel better	
Was accepting/nonjudgmental	Made judgmental comments OR facial expressions	Did not express judgment but did not demonstrate respect	Made comments and expressions that demonstrated respect	
Used words you understood and/or explained jargon	Consistently used jargon WITHOUT further explanation	Sometimes used jargon AND did not explain it	Explained jargon when used OR avoided completely	

Education and counseling	Not done	Partially done	Well done	Comments
Asked questions to see what you understood (checked your understanding)	Did not check for understanding	Asked if patient had any questions BUT did not check for understanding	Assessed understanding by checking in throughout	
Provided clear explanations/information	Gave confusing/no explanations—made it impossible to understand	Info was somewhat clear BUT still led to some difficulty in understanding	Provided small bits of info AND summarized to make sure clear	
Collaborated with you in identifying possible next steps/plan	Told patient next steps/plan (OR no next steps/plan)	Told patient next steps THEN asked patient's views	Discussed options THEN mutually developed plan	

Organization and time management	Not done	Partially done	Well done	Comments
Managed time effectively	Paced the encounter poorly; did not manage time well	Paced the encounter, managed time to cover most of what needed to be covered	Paced the encounter very well; managed time so that visit seemed complete	

RESIDENT CASE-SPECIFIC SKILLS

Assessing history	Not done	Partially done	Well done	*Comments*
Asked for *name and date of birth*	Did not ask	Asked for either name only or date of birth only	Asked for name and date of birth	
Asked about *past medical problems*	Did not ask patient past medical problems	Asked if patient has any past medical problems but not specific	Asked a comprehensive past medical history—including meds, allergies	
Asked about *alcohol use*	Did not ask	Asked about BUT NOT quantity or frequency	Asked about AND assessed quantity and frequency	
Asked about *drug use*	Did not ask	Asked about BUT NOT quantity or frequency	Asked about AND assessed quantity and frequency	
Asked about *smoking*	Did not ask	Asked about BUT NOT quantity or frequency	Asked about AND assessed quantity and frequency	
Asked about *work history* and *educational level*	Did not ask	Asked about current job but not work history and/or educational level	Asked about all	
Asked about *social and family support*	Did not ask	Asked questions about family/friends	Identified access to support	
Asked about *family medical history*	Did not ask	Asked generally but not specifically	Obtained a full family medical history	
Asked about *depression*	Did not ask	Asked generally about depression but did not use the PHQ-2	Asked about depression using at least the PHQ-2 (asked about *lack of interest* AND *mood*)	
Offered *HIV* screening	Did not offer	Offered test (learned that you are HIV-negative)		
Asked about *tetanus* and *other immunizations*	Did not ask	Asked about one vaccine	Asked about more than one vaccines	

YES	Not sure	*Review of systems* Asked about...	YES		Not sure	*Physical exam*
☐	Not sure	*Skin* Rash, itching, pigmentation, dryness, hair growth or loss	☐ PCA	☐ Intern	Not sure	*Vital signs* Measured blood pressure, took pulse
			☐		Not sure	*Washed Hands Before Exam*
☐	Not sure	*Eyes/ears/nose/mouth/throat* Vision, hearing, throat pain, headache	☐ *Please circle*		Not sure	*Eyes/Ears/Nose/Mouth/Throat* Inspected
☐	Not sure	*Cardiovascular* Chest pain, palpitations, shortness of breath, walking	☐		Not sure	*Heart* Listened
			☐		Not sure	*Checked extremities* Felt pulses, inspected hands/feet
☐	Not sure	*Respiratory* Shortness of breath, wheezing	☐		Not sure	*Lungs* Listened, palpated, and/or percussed
☐	Not sure	*Musculoskeletal* Pain, swelling, redness/heat muscles/joint; range of motion	☐		Not sure	*Strength/range of motion* Inspected and tested muscles and joints

YES	Not sure	*Review of systems* Asked about...	YES	Not sure	*Physical exam*
☐	Not Sure	*OB/GYN* Pregnancy, menstruation, last pap smear, gyn health	☐	Not Sure	*Abdomen* Inspected, listened, palpated, and/or percussed
☐	Not Sure	*Gastrointestinal* Bowel movements, pain, swallowing, appetite	☐	Not Sure	*OTHER* _____
☐	Not Sure	*Allergic/immunologic/lymphatic/endocrine* Reactions to drugs, food, insects, skin rashes; trouble breathing; anemia; lymph nodes	☐	Not Sure	*OTHER* _____

Patient education	**Not done**	**Partially done**	**Well done**	*Comments*
Assessed your *understanding of asthma*	Did not assess	Obtained a full history of your personal experience of asthma OR asked what you know about the condition	Fully explored both your personal experiences of asthma and understanding of the condition	
Assessed your *understanding of asthma medications*	Did not asses understanding	Told you how asthma medications work without assessing understanding	Assessed understanding and corrected misinformation	
Checked/demonstrated *inhaler technique*	Didn't address inhaler technique	Demonstrated or explained correct use but didn't check inhaler technique	Checked your technique and demonstrated correct use	
Recommended that you use the *controller/ preventive inhaler (Flovent)* daily for better symptom management	Didn't recommend	Suggested that you should use the Flovent inhaler daily	Gave a clear and direct recommendation that you should use the Flovent and explained how it would better manage symptoms	
Recommended short course of *prednisone (oral steroids)*	Did not recommend	Recommended several days of steroids		
Recommended that you use your *inhaler with a spacer*	Did not recommend	Recommended that you use spacer		
Gave a list of prescribed medications	Did not give the list of medications	Gave list but did not discuss medications prescribed	Gave the list and fully explained medications prescribed	
Labs/referrals ordered ___ Respiratory therapy referral ___Other: _____	Ordered no labs	Offered labs/referrals but did not explain which ones and rationale behind decision	Offered labs, explained choice and rationale for labs and discusses follow up of results	

Made which of the following	**Yes**	**NS**	**Health maintenance recommendation**	*Comments*
health maintenance recommendations:	☐	Not sure	Take preventive medication (Flovent)	
	☐	Not sure	*Other:* _____	

Counseling (Man and Tx)	Not done	Partially done	Well done	Comments
Reviewed *plan* with you	Did not review summation of visit and plan	Reviewed plan but did not assess ability/willingness to comply	Reviewed plan, assessed ability, willingness to comply	
Asked you what *further questions* you have	Did not ask	Asked about questions but in a brisk manner, didn't allow sufficient time	Asked you what further questions you had in a way that invited questions	
Gave information about *follow-up and further contact* with MD	Did not address	Addressed follow-up but was not specific	Specifically addressed follow-up, setting time, and person	
Helped you understand how to *navigate* the system in order to *follow through* on next steps	Did not help navigate the system	Partially explained how system works in terms of next steps (blood work etc.)	Fully explained the process and how to navigate the system	

PATIENT CENTEREDNESS/SATISFACTION

The resident ...	Not done	Partially done	Well done	Comments
Answered or addressed all my *questions*/concerns	Only answered/ addressed a few of the most central	Answered/addressed many of my questions/concerns	Answered/addressed all of my questions/concerns	
Took a *personal interest* in me; treated me as a *person*	Did not see me as a person	Viewed me as a person, but did not take personal interest	Took an active personal interest in me	
Gave me *enough information*	Not given much info at all	I was given some information but I still had questions	I was given all the information I wanted/needed	
Made you feel like had *enough time* (not rushed)	Did not have enough time; visit felt rushed	Mostly had enough time (visit a bit rushed); felt some time pressure	Felt no real-time pressures; covered most w/out pressure	

ACTIVATING THE PATIENT

This encounter....	Not done	Partially done	Well done	Comments
This encounter helped me to understand the nature and causes of asthma	Did not help me understand	Helped me understand some things but not everything	Helped me fully understand what happened	
After the encounter, *I understood how to manage my asthma in the future* (including how medications work and how to use them)	I did not learn about asthma management	I found out about some of the treatment options	I left with a clear treatment and management plan	
This visit made me feel *confident I can keep asthma interfering* too much with my life	Did not affect my confidence	Helped me feel more confident that I could keep asthma with life	Helped me feel very confident that I could keep asthma from interfering with my life	
Because of this encounter, I am *confident I can figure out solutions* if something new comes up	Did not affect my confidence	Helped me feel somewhat confident that I could deal with new issues	Helped me feel quite confident that I could deal with new issues	

OVERALL RECOMMENDATIONS

Would you recommend this doctor to a friend or family member for his/her....

Communication/interpersonal skills?	Not recommend	Recommend with reservations	Recommend	Highly recommend
Medical competence? Application of medical knowledge	Not recommend	Recommend with reservations	Recommend	Highly recommend
Professionalism? Accountable, respectful, sensitive and/or responsive, compassionate	Not recommend	Recommend with reservations	Recommend	Highly recommend

Would you recommend this *clinic* to a friend if they needed primary care?

Not recommend	Recommend with reservations	Recommend	Highly recommend
Please explain your choice (comment on anything you feel is relevant including the facility, staff, waiting area, and time spent waiting):			

DETECTION

Do you think this physician recognized that you were a Standardized Patient?

No	Yes	*If yes, explain why*

What materials did you receive during this visit?

Yes	Materials
☐	Lab orders
☐	Health education pamphlets/information
☐	Contact information
☐	Follow-up appointment slip
☐	Hand written note, diagram, explanation
☐	Spacer or inhaler
☐	*Other:* _____

Please use the following timeline to depict the sequence and timing of the visit.

Divide the timeline into four major segments of the case: History gathering (HG), physical examination (PE), counseling about Asthma and medication (ASTH), report to preceptor (PRE), health recommendations (HR). Place them in the same order as in the visit and do your best to represent the portion of the visit that was spent on each. If time during the visit was spent on other issues please describe and put on the timeline too!

Start   End

Did anything unusual or remarkable happen during (or related to) your encounter?

OVERALL COMMENTS (additional remarks, factors affecting your score, etc):

Appendix P
Other Resources

Station Development

- Search MEDLINE (http://www.ncbi.nlm.nih.gov/pubmed) and the Internet for articles describing OSCEs and OSCE stations.
- MedEdPortal (www.mededportal.org) provides a peer-reviewed collection of free educational resources including cases and OSCE stations.
- OSCE exam preparation books (e.g., Hurley 2005) and Web sites (e.g., OSCE Home: www.oscehome.com/) contain station examples.
- Consider non-OSCE Clinical Vignettes that can be converted into OSCE cases.
- The Association for Standardized Patient Educators (ASPE: www.aspeducators.org) includes a virtual library with resources for station development (some resources require membership in the organization).
- Professional listservs/blogs; may require registration but can provide opportunities to access expertise and resources worldwide: SP-Trainer (mailman2.u.washington.edu/mailman/listinfo/sp-trainer), the official ASPE listserv; DR ED (list.msu.edu/cgi-bin/wa?A0=dr-ed), an international general listserv focusing on medical education; eGroups of the Society for Simulation in Healthcare (www.ssih.org).

Standardized Patient Recruitment and Training

- The Association for Standardized Patient Educators (ASPE) holds annual conferences and gives out annual project awards which provide further resources (e.g., feedback training, recruitment, and training of multicultural SPs). Their Web site (www.aspeducators.org) includes a searchable bibliography organized in the following sections: Overviews of SP Use; Project or Program Evaluation; SPs in Teaching Exercises; OSCEs; Measurement Tools; Influence of being an SP on the SP/Special Populations of SPs; Models and Computers for Simulation.
- Wallace (2007) provides an excellent in-depth resource for SP coaching.

Educational Research and Psychometrics

- Look for university courses on educational measurement in departments of education or psychology.
- The Association of American Medical Colleges (AAMC) runs a number of relevant training programs, such as the Medical Education Research Certificate (MERC) (www.aamc.org/members/gea/merc) through their Group on Educational Affairs (GEA).
- Consult the Foundation for Advancement of International Medical Education and Research (FAIMER: www.faimer.org) for fellowship opportunities.

S. Zabar et al. (eds.), *Objective Structured Clinical Examinations*,
DOI 10.1007/978-1-4614-3749-9, © Springer Science+Business Media New York 2013

References

Articles, Reports and Books

Accreditation Council for Graduate Medical Education (ACGME) Outcomes Project and the American Board of Medical Specialties (ABMS) Joint Initiative. Toolbox of Assessment Methods. ACGME, ABMS, 2000.

Accreditation Council for Graduate Medical Education. ACGME Core Competencies. ACGME;2001. Available online: www.acgme.org/acwebsite/RRC_280/280_corecomp.asp. Accessed 1 Apr 2012.

Aeder L, Altshuler L, Kachur EK, Barrett S, Hilfer A, Koepfer S, Schaeffer H, Shelov SP. The "Culture OSCE"—introducing a formative assessment into a postgraduate program. Educ Health. 2007;20:11.

Adamo G. Simulated and standardized patients in OSCEs: achievements and challenges 1992–2003. Med Teach. 2003;25:262–70.

Altshuler L, Kachur EK. A culture OSCE: teaching residents to bridge different worlds. Acad Med. 2001;76:514.

Altshuler L, Kachur E, Krinshpun S, Sullivan D. Genetics objective structured clinical exams at the Maimonides infants & Children's hospital of Brooklyn, New York. Acad Med. 2008;83:1088–93.

Anderson MB, Kassebaum DG. Proceedings of the AAMC consensus conference on the use of standardized patients in the teaching and evaluation of clinical skills. Acad Med. 1993;68:437–83.

Association of American Medical Colleges (AAMC) Medical School Objectives Project. Report I: Learning Objectives for Medical Student Education—Guidelines for Medical Schools. AAMC, 1998.

Barrows HS, Abrahamson S. The programmed patient: a technique for appraising student performance in clinical neurology. J Med Educ. 1964;39:802–5.

Boulet JR, De Champlain AF, McKinley DW. Setting defensible performance standards on OSCEs and standardized patient examinations. Med Teach. 2003;25:245–9.

Boulet JR, Smee SM, Dillon GF, Gimpel JR. The use of standardized patient assessments for certification and licensure decisions. Simul Healthc. 2009;4:35–42.

Bowen JL. Educational strategies to promote clinical diagnostic reasoning. N Engl J Med. 2006;355:2217–25.

Carney P, Ward D. Using unannounced standardized patients to assess the HIV preventive practices of family nurse practitioners and family physicians. Nurse Pract. 1998;23(2):56–8. 63, 67–8 passim.

Casebeer L, Klapow J, Centor R. An intervention to increase physicians' use of adherence-enhancing strategies in managing hypercholesterolemic patients. Acad Med. 1999;74:1334–9.

Chander B, Kule R, Baiocco P, Chokhavatia S, Kotler D, Poles M, Zabar S, Gillespie C, Ark T, Weinshel E. Teaching the competencies: using objective structured clinical encounters for gastroenterology fellows. Clin Gastroenterol Hepatol. 2009;7:509–14.

Cleland J, Arnold R, Chesser A. Failing finals is often a surprise for the student but not the teacher: identifying difficulties and supporting students with academic difficulties. Med Teach. 2005;27:504–8.

Culver J, Bowen D, Reynolds S, Pinsky LE, Press N, Burke W. Breast cancer risk communication: assessment of primary care physicians by standardized patients. Genet Med. 2009;11:735–41.

Cumming AD, Ross MT. Tuning Project (medicine)—learning outcomes/competences for undergraduate medical education in Europe. Edinburgh: The University of Edinburgh; 2008. Available online: www.tuning-medicine.com. Accessed 1 Apr 2012.

Croskerry P. The importance of cognitive errors in diagnosis and strategies to minimize them. Acad Med. 2003;78:775–80.

Downing SA, Tekian A, Yudkowsky R. Procedures for establishing defensible absolute passing scores on performance examinations in health professions education. Teach Learn Med. 2006;18:50–7.

Epstein R, Franks P, Shields CG, Meldrum SC, Miller KN, Campbell TL, Fiscella K. Patient-centered communication and diagnostic testing. Ann Fam Med. 2005;3:415–21.

Glassman P, Luck J, O'Gara E, Peabody J. Using standardized patients to measure quality: evidence from the literature and a prospective study. Jt Comm J Qual Improv. 2000;26:644–53.

Harden RM, Stevenson M, Downie WW, Wilson GM. Assessment of clinical competence using objective structured examination. Br Med J. 1975;1:447–51.

Harris G. New for aspiring doctors, the people skills test. The New York Times. 10 Jul 2011.

Hatchett P, Haun C, Goldenhar L. Training standardized patients to give feedback to medical trainees: The state of the art. ASPE Project Awards, 2004. Available online at: www.aspeducators.org/aspe-project-awards.php. Accessed 1 Apr 2012.

Hauer KE, Ciccone A, Henzel TR, Katsufrakis P, Miller SH, Norcross WA, Papadakis MA, Irby DM. Remediation of the deficiencies of physicians across the continuum from medical school to practice: a thematic review of the literature. Acad Med. 2009;84:1822–32.

Hodges B. The objective structured clinical examination: a socio-history. Koeln, Germany: LAP Lambert Academic Publishing; 2009.

Hodges B, McIlroy JH. Analytic global OSCE ratings are sensitive to level of training. Med Educ. 2003;37(11):1012–6.

Hurley KF. OSCE and clinical skills handbook. Toronto, ON: Elsevier Health Sciences; 2005.

Institute of Medicine (IOM) Board on Health Care Services Committee on the Health Professions Summit. In: Greiner A, Knebel E, editors.

Health professions education: a bridge to quality. National Academies Press, 2003. Available online at: www.iom.edu/Reports/2003/Health-Professions-Education-A-Bridge-to-Quality.aspx. Accessed 1 Apr 2012.

Jefferies A, Simmons B, Tabak D, McIlroy JH, Lee KS, Roukema H, Skidmore M. Using an objective structured clinical examination (OSCE) to assess multiple physician competencies in postgraduate training. Med Teach. 2007;29:183–91.

Kachur E. OSCEs in the US. In: Otaki J, editor. Theory and practice of the OSCE. Tokyo: Shinohara Shuppan Shinsha; 2007. p. 204–17 [Japanese].

Kachur EK, Green S, Dennis C. Written comments on Objective Structured Clinical Exam (OSCE) rating forms: an exploratory study. Teach Learn Med. 1990;2:225–31.

Kalet A, Earp JA, Kowlowitz V. How well do faculty evaluate the interviewing skills of medical students? J Gen Intern Med. 1992;7(5):499–505.

Kilminster S, Roberts T. Standard setting for OSCEs: trial of borderline approach. Adv Health Sci Educ Theory Pract. 2004;9:201–9.

Kogan J, Holmboe E, Hauer K. Tools for direct observation and assessment of clinical skills of medical trainees: a systematic review. JAMA. 2009;302:1316–26.

Krumer A, Muijijens A, Jansen K, Dusman H, Tan L, van der Vleuten C. Comparison of a rational and an empirical standard setting procedure for an OSCE. Med Educ. 2003;37:132–9.

Lamont CT, Hennen BK. The use of simulated patients in a certification examination in family medicine. J Med Educ. 1972;47:789–95.

Morrison LJ, Barrows HS. Educational impact of the Macy Consortia: regional development of clinical practice examinations. Final report of the EMPAC Project, 1998.

Newble DI, Hoare J, Sheldrake PF. The selection and training of examiners for clinical examinations. Med Educ. 1980;14:345–9.

Norcini J, Anderson B, Bollela V, Burch V, Costa MJ, Duvivier R, Galbraith R, Hays R, Kent A, Perrott V, Roberts T. Criteria for good assessment: consensus statement and recommendations from the Ottawa 2010 conference. Med Teach. 2011;33:206–14.

Ozuah P, Reznik M. Residents' asthma communication skills in announced versus unannounced standardized patient exercises. Ambul Pediatr. 2007;7:445–8.

Ozuah P, Reznik M. Using unannounced standardized patients to assess residents' competency in asthma severity classification. Ambul Pediatr. 2008a;8:139–42.

Ozuah P, Reznik M. Using unannounced standardized patients to assess residents' professionalism. Med Educ. 2008b;42:532–43.

Parish SJ, Ramaswamy M, Stein MR, Kachur EK, Arnsten JH. Teaching about substance abuse with Objective Structured Clinical Exams. J Gen Intern Med. 2006;21:453–9.

Peabody J, Luck J, Glassman P, Dresselhaus TR, Lee M. Comparison of vignettes, standardized patients, and chart abstraction: a prospective validation study of 3 methods for measuring quality. JAMA. 2000;283:1715–22.

Peabody J, Luck J, Jain S, Bertenthal D, Glassman P. Assessing the accuracy of administrative data in health information systems. Med Care. 2004;42:1066–72.

Petrusa ER, Guckian JC, Perkowski LC. A multiple station objective clinical evaluation. Res Med Educ. 1984;23:211–6.

Pinsky L, Wipf J. A picture is worth a thousand words: practical use of videotape in teaching. J Gen Intern Med. 2000;15:805–10.

Poenaru D, Morales D, Richards A, O'Connor HM. Running an objective structured clinical examination on a shoestring budget. Am J Surg. 1997;173:538–41.

Quirk M. Intuition and metacognition in medical education: keys to developing expertise. New York: Springer; 2006.

Rethans J, Gorter S, Bokken L, Morrison L. Unannounced standardized patients in real practice: a systematic literature review. Med Educ. 2007;41:537–49.

Reznick RK, Smee S, Baumber JS, Cohen R, Rothman A, Blackmore D, Berard M. Guidelines for estimating the real cost of an objective structured clinical examination. Acad Med. 1993;68:513–7.

Sadler DR. Interpretations of criteria-based assessment and grading in higher education. Asses Eval High Educ. 2005;30:175–94.

Sayer M, Chaput de Saintonge M, Evans D, Wood D. Support for students with academic difficulties. Med Educ. 2002;36:643–50.

Schwartz RW, Witzke DB, Donnelly MB, Stratton T, Blue AV, Sloan DA. Assessing residents' clinical performance: cumulative results of a four-year study with the Objective Structured Clinical Examination. Surgery. 1998;124:307–12.

Segal SS, Giordani B, Gillum LH, Johnson N. The academic support program at the University of Michigan School of Medicine. Acad Med. 1999;74:383–5.

Shah R, Edgar D, Evans B. Measuring clinical practice. Ophthalmic Physiol Opt. 2007;27:113–25.

Silverman J, Kurtz S, Draper JH. Skills for communicating with patients. 2nd ed. Oxford, UK: Radcliffe Publishing; 2005.

Stillman PL, Brown D, Redfield D, Sabers D. Construct validation of the Arizona Clinical Interviewing Rating Scale. Educ Psychol Meas. 1977;37:1031–78.

Sutnick AI, Stillman PL, Norcini JJ, Friedman M, Regan MB, Williams RG, Kachur EK, Haggerty MA, Wilson MP. ECFMG assessment of clinical competence of graduates of foreign medical schools. JAMA. 1993;270:1041–5.

Tamblyn RM, Klass DJ, Schnabl GK, Kopelow ML. The accuracy of standardized patient presentation. Med Educ. 1991;25:100–9.

Wallace P. Coaching standardized patients for Use in the assessment of clinical competence. New York: Springer; 2007.

Wayne State School of Medicine Standardized Patient Program. Case Development Blueprint. Wayne State School of Medicine, 2011.

Yedidia M, Gillespie C, Kachur E, Schwartz M, Ockene J, Chepaitis A, Snyder C, Lazare A, Lipkin Jr M. Effect of communications training on medical student performance. JAMA. 2003;290:1157–65.

Zabar S, Ark T, Gillespie C, Hsieh A, Kalet A, Kachur E, Manko J, Regan L. Can unannounced standardized patients assess professionalism and communication skills in the emergency department? Acad Emerg Med. 2009;16:915–8.

Zabar S, Hanley K, Kachur E, Stevens D, Schwartz MD, Pearlman E, Adams J, Felix K, Lipkin Jr M, Kalet A. "Oh! She doesn't speak English!" Assessing resident competence in managing linguistic and cultural barriers. J Gen Intern Med. 2006;21:510–3.

Zabar S, Hanley K, Stevens D, Kalet A, Schwartz M, Pearlman E, Brenner J, Kachur EK, Lipkin M. Measuring the competence of residents as teachers. J Gen Intern Med. 2004;19(5 Pt 2):530–3.

Websites

American Association of Colleges of Osteopathic Medicine (AECOM). www.aacom.org. Accessed 1 Apr 2012

Association of American Medical Colleges (AAMC). www.aamc.org. Accessed 1 Apr 2012

Association of Standardized Patient Educators (ASPE). www.aspeducators.org. Accessed 1 Apr 2012

Centers for Disease Control (CDC). Epi Info 7. wwwn.cdc.gov/epiinfo. Accessed 1 Apr 2012

The College of Family Physicians of Canada. Family Medicine Examination. www.cfpc.ca/FMExam/. Accessed 1 Apr 2012

Federation of State Medical Boards (FSMB) and the National Board of Medical Examiners (NBME). United States Medical Licensing Examination – Step 2 CS (Clinical Skills). www.usmle.org/step-2-cs/. Accessed 1 Apr 2012

Foundation for Advancement of International Medical Education and Research (FAIMER). www.faimer.org. Accessed 1 Apr 2012

Medical Council of Canada (MCC). Qualifying Examination Part II. www.mcc.ca/en/exams/qe2/. Accessed 1 Apr 2012

MedEdPORTAL. www.mededportal.org. Accessed 1 Apr 2012

MedInfo Consulting. OSCE Home. www.oscehome.com. Accessed 1 Apr 2012

National Board of Medical Examiners (NBME). www.nbme.org. Accessed 1 Apr 2012

National Board of Osteopathic Medical Examiners (NBOME). COMPLEX L2-PE FAQ and Information. www.nbome.org/comlex-pe.asp?m=can Accessed 1 Apr 2012.

Royal College of Physicians and Surgeons of Canada. The CanMEDS 2005 Physician Competency Framework. http://rcpsc.medical.org/canmeds/CanMEDS2005/. Accessed 1 Apr 2012

Society for Simulation in Healthcare (SSH). www.ssih.org. Accessed 1 Apr 2012

U.S. Department of Education. Family Educational Rights and Privacy Act. www2.ed.gov/policy/gen/guid/fpco/ferpa/index.html. Accessed 1 Apr 2012

U.S. Department of Health & Human Services. Understanding Health Information Privacy. www.hhs.gov/ocr/privacy/hipaa/understanding/index.html. Accessed 1 Apr 2012

Vroman Systems, Inc. FormSite. www.formsite.com. Accessed 1 Apr 2012

Index